The First Episode of Psychosis

The First Episode of Psychosis

A Guide for Patients and Their Families

Michael T. Compton, M.D., M.P.H.

and

Beth Broussard, M.P.H., C.H.E.S

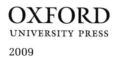

OXFORD
UNIVERSITY PRESS

2009

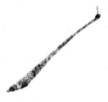

OXFORD
UNIVERSITY PRESS

Oxford University Press, Inc., publishes works that further
Oxford University's objective of excellence
in research, scholarship, and education.

Oxford New York
Auckland Cape Town Dar es Salaam Hong Kong Karachi
Kuala Lumpur Madrid Melbourne Mexico City Nairobi
New Delhi Shanghai Taipei Toronto

With offices in
Argentina Austria Brazil Chile Czech Republic France Greece
Guatemala Hungary Italy Japan Poland Portugal Singapore
South Korea Switzerland Thailand Turkey Ukraine Vietnam

Published by Oxford University Press, Inc.
198 Madison Avenue, New York, New York 10016
www.oup.com

Oxford is a registered trademark of Oxford University Press

Library of Congress Cataloging-in-Publication Data
Compton, Michael T.
The first episode of psychosis : a guide for patients and their families / Michael T.
Compton and Beth Broussard.
    p. cm.
Includes bibliographical references
ISBN 978-0-19-537249-6 (alk. paper)   1. Psychoses— Popular works.
I. Broussard, Beth. II. Title.
RC512.C58 2009
616.89—dc22
2008044049

9 8 7 6 5 4 3
Printed in the United States of America
on acid-free paper

Acknowledgments

We are extremely grateful to our colleagues in The ACES Project (Atlanta Cohort on the Early course of Schizophrenia), who have been enormously supportive as we developed this book. In fact, many of our team members, listed by name in the following pages, generously volunteered to help in writing initial drafts of chapters. We are very fortunate to have such hard-working, dedicated, enthusiastic, and fun coworkers, and we look forward to continuing our research and clinical work involving first-episode patients and their families with this great team.

We are also very appreciative of the numerous expert collaborators who reviewed specific chapters, provided very helpful critiques and advice, and encouraged our work on this project. Again, they are listed by name in the pages that follow. We admire their research, clinical programs, and dedication to patients and families, all of which are done with a spirit of collaboration and hope. It is this sense of optimism and recovery-orientation, so characteristic of the emerging early intervention model, that we hope to pass along in this book. We also appreciate the initial feedback and support of Dr. Jean Addington and Dr. Patrick McGorry of the International Early Phychosis Association.

We also thank a number of people important in our lives who have tolerated the long hours we spent on developing this book. Their unwavering support was essential to its completion. We especially thank certain individuals who gave of their time and provided valuable reviews of the entire manuscript, including Sandy Goulding, Claire Ramsay, and Kendrick Hogan. At Oxford University Press, we are greatly indebted to Sarah Harrington for her ongoing encouragement, support, and assistance. She kindly answered countless questions and openly considered our big and small ideas during the book's evolution. We greatly appreciate the opportunity to visit the art therapy program at Skyland Trail, an innovative treatment and recovery center in Atlanta, Georgia, and recipient of the 2004 Gold Achievement Award given by the American Psychiatric Association. They generously welcomed our idea for a cover image created by an individual in recovery and assisted us in finding the perfect piece for the front of the book. We also thank the artist for allowing us the opportunity to express the same message on the book's front cover that he strives to promote in his inspired work.

Finally, and most importantly, we would like to acknowledge our patients and their family members, who inspired us to write this book for them, and who continue to teach us about the complex syndrome of psychosis. We hope that our efforts will be helpful in their path towards recovery after the first episode of psychosis.

MTC & BB

The ACES Project Team Members Who Assisted with Initial Chapter Development

Erin M. Bergner, MPH
Tandrea Carter, PhD
Victoria H. Chien, BA
Michelle L. Esterberg, MPH, MA
Lauren Franz, MBChB, MPH
Sandra M. Goulding, MPH
Amy S. Leiner, PhD
Claire E. Ramsay, MPH
Kevin D. Tessner, PhD
Hanan D. Trotman, MA

International Collaborators Who Provided Expert Reviews of Specific Chapters

Jean Addington, PhD
Alberta Centennial Mental
    Health Research Chair
    and Novartis Chair in
    Schizophrenia Research
Professor
University of Calgary
Department of Psychiatry
Calgary, Alberta, Canada

**Matthew R. Broome, MRCPsych,
    PhD**
Associate Clinical Professor
    of Psychiatry and Honorary
    Consultant Psychiatrist in
    Early Intervention
Warwick Medical School
University of Warwick

Health Sciences Research
    Institute
Coventry,
United Kingdom

Kristin Cadenhead, MD
Professor
University of California San
    Diego
Department of Psychiatry
La Jolla, California, California
United States

Cheryl Corcoran, MD
Florence Irving Assistant
Professor of Clinical Psychiatry
Columbia University Medical
    Center

Director, Center of Prevention
and Evaluation
New York State Psychiatric
Institute
New York, New York,
United States

Robert E. Drake, MD, PhD
Professor of Psychiatry and of
Community and Family
Medicine
Dartmouth Medical School
Director, Dartmouth Dual
Diagnosis Center, Dartmouth
Psychiatric Research Center
Co-Director, Dartmouth
Supported Employment
Center, Dartmouth
Psychiatric Research
Center
Hanover, New Hampshire,
United States

Jane Edwards, PhD
Deputy Clinical Director
ORYGEN Youth Health
Melbourne, Victoria,
Australia

Jacqueline Maus Feldman, MD
Patrick H. Linton Professor of
Psychiatry
Director, Division of Public
Psychiatry
University of Alabama at
Birmingham School of
Medicine
Department of Psychiatry and
Behavioral Neurobiology

UAB Community Psychiatry
Program
Birmingham, Alabama,
United States

Philip D. Harvey, PhD
Professor
Emory University School of
Medicine
Department of Psychiatry and
Behavioral Sciences
Atlanta, Georgia,
United States

Srividya N. Iyer, PhD
Program Coordinator
McGill University
Department of Psychiatry
Douglas Mental Health
University Institute
Prevention and Early Intervention
Program for Psychoses (PEPP)
Montreal, Quebec,
Canada

Inge Joa, MHS, RN
Administrative Coordinator
Stavanger University Hospital,
Department of Psychiatry
TIPS—Regional Centre for
Clinical Research in
Psychosis
Stavanger, Norway

Anthony Jorm, PhD, DSc
Professorial Fellow
University of Melbourne
ORYGEN Research Centre
Melbourne, Victoria,
Australia

Nadine J. Kaslow, PhD
Professor and Chief
　Psychologist
Emory University School of
　Medicine
Department of Psychiatry and
　Behavioral Sciences
Atlanta, Georgia,
United States

Eóin Killackey, DPsych
Senior Research Fellow and
　Clinical Psychologist
University of Melbourne
Department of Psychology
ORYGEN Research
　Centre
Melbourne, Victoria,
Australia

Brian Kirkpatrick, MD, MSPH
Vice Chair
Medical College of
　Georgia
Department of Psychiatry and
　Health Behavior
Augusta, Georgia,
United States

Betty Kitchener, BA, MNse
Lecturer
University of Melbourne
Department of Psychiatry
ORYGEN Research Centre
Mental Health First Aid
Melbourne, Victoria,
Australia

Tor K. Larsen, MD, PhD
Professor
University of Bergen
Department of Psychiatry
Stavanger University
　Hospital
Department of Psychiatry
Stavanger,
Norway

**Ashok Malla, MBBS, FRCPC,
　MRCPsych**
Canada Research Chair in
　Early Psychosis
Professor
McGill University
Department of Psychiatry
Douglas Mental Health
　University Institute
Director, Clinical Research
　Division
Director, Prevention and Early
　intervention Program for
　Psychoses (PEPP)
Montreal, Quebec,
Canada

Ross M. G. Norman, PhD
Professor
University of Western
　Ontario
Schulich School of
　Medcine
Departments of Psychiatry,
　and Epidemiology and
　Biostatistics
London, Ontario,
Canada

Elaine F. Walker, PhD
Samuel Candler Dobbs
    Professor of Psychology and
    Neuroscience
Emory University
Graduate School of Arts and
    Sciences
Department of Psychology
Atlanta, Georgia,
United States

Amy C. Watson, PhD
Assistant Professor
University of Illinois at Chicago
Jane Addams College of Social
    Work
Chicago, Illinois,
United States

Foreword

In psychiatry, and the broader field of mental health, there have been remarkable changes in the past 20 years in terms of attitudes and knowledge, as well as in access to care and quality of care for people with schizophrenia and other psychotic illnesses. This has been particularly true for those experiencing a first episode of psychosis. The revolutionary work of some exceptionally dedicated researchers and clinicians has had an unparalleled impact on the mental health field in terms of early intervention, such that this focus has become a worldwide movement with programs and services being developed on every continent. This is an exciting time for improving the lives of people affected by psychosis. Yet, a lot more work has to be done because specialized care for a first episode of psychosis is not always available.

Regardless of whether treatment occurs in a specialized first-episode program or in the local mental health center, the first episode of psychosis can be a frightening and bewildering period for young people and their families. Usually with no previous experience to guide them, the young person and his or her family often feel overwhelmed. Access to care and treatment are oftentimes delayed, and people may not even know where to turn for help. Clinics may be busy and, despite the best intentions, may not always help patients and their families really understand the illness and the complicated issues of prognosis, treatment, and outcome.

The authors of this book, Dr. Michael Compton and Ms. Beth Broussard, have put together a remarkable and much needed guide, based on their own clinical and health education expertise grounded in research conducted by The ACES Project, led by Dr. Compton at Emory University and Grady Health System in Atlanta, Georgia, United States. With assistance from their coworkers and collaboration from a group of international experts, they have written a guide that will help young people experiencing a first psychotic episode and their families through the many crises, stages, turning points, and outcomes of their episode. This book promotes learning about the illness and treatments and addresses the multitude of questions, issues, and concerns that typically arise. This guide should be accessible to all patients and families regardless of where they may be seeking help.

Jean Addington, PhD
President, International Early Psychosis Association

Preface

What is happening? What are these voices? These odd and unusual ideas? What is causing it? Who can help? What will the doctors do? Is this treatment really necessary? What should I do next? Is this curable? Will it come back? What will people think? How can our family cope? What should I do if things get worse at home?

These are some of the many questions that often go through the minds of people experiencing psychosis and their family members. An episode of psychosis can be frightening. It can be confusing. It can even seem like life is changing forever.

We work closely with people who are experiencing psychosis for the first time and with their families. We know the many questions that come up. We want to help. We wrote this book to try to answer these questions and many more. As a psychiatrist and researcher specializing in schizophrenia and related psychotic disorders, and a health educator specializing in mental health literacy, we have brought together our expertise and understanding of psychosis. We have aimed to provide readers with a complete guide explaining everything they need to know during this critical time of initial evaluation and treatment.

This book is meant to help readers through a very difficult, painful, and confusing time. We expect that people reading this book will include both patients and their family members. Throughout the book, we use certain terms to help with the ease of reading because of the range of our audience. We often use the term *patient* for simplicity. The word typically refers to a person who is seeking care from a doctor. Other terms may be more appropriate nowadays, like *client* or *consumer*, and we recognize that the term *patient* is problematic for some people. But for simplicity and ease of writing and reading, we often refer to individuals experiencing psychosis who are seeking help as *patients*. We also frequently use the term *family* or *family members* for simplicity. Here, we mean not only immediate relatives, like mothers, fathers, brothers, and sisters, but also extended family members, friends, significant others, and other important people in the lives of patients. Similarly, we sometimes use the word *doctor* rather than the more general term *mental health professional*. Although a variety of mental health professionals, like psychiatrists, psychologists, nurses, social workers, counselors, and others are involved in the care of people with psychosis, we sometimes use *doctor* for simplicity, especially in chapters dealing with diagnosis and medications. Please forgive us for the use of these terms if they do not seem to fit. After much discussion, we have chosen to use them at points in the book because of our main focus on readability and simplicity as well as on important concepts and information.

Another wording concern that we would like to point out is that we often use the terms *first episode of psychosis* and *first-episode psychosis*. This refers to the initial period of experiencing psychotic symptoms and the mental health evaluation and treatment for this episode of psychosis. For some people, this becomes the first of several or many episodes of psychosis, in which case the use of the term *first episode* is truly warranted. However, we do not mean to suggest that everyone who has a first episode of psychosis will necessarily go on to have future episodes of psychosis. For some people, the symptoms clear up with treatment. These people achieve long-term remission and recovery without later episodes. We also sometimes use *early psychosis* to mean roughly the same as the first episode of psychosis.

In each chapter, there are bold words and phrases. These words are ones that we think are important and need to be further explained. Definitions for each of these words are included in the Glossary at the end of the book. There also are collaborators listed for most chapters. These individuals are international experts in that chapter's topic who helped to make sure that the information provided was the best and most useful to readers.

We want to provide you with the information that you need to begin a path towards recovery or to go about helping a loved one towards recovery. We invite you to read this book and gather from it whatever information is helpful to you. The book is divided into three parts, each one building on the next as you learn more about the first episode of psychosis.

Part I, Answering Your Basic Questions, focuses on explaining the basics of psychosis, including what it is, symptoms, different diagnoses associated with it, and possible causes. In Chapter 1, What Is Psychosis?, we define and demystify psychosis. This chapter was initially developed with assistance from Victoria Chien, BA, and Michelle Esterberg, MPH, MA. Cheryl Corcoran, MD, and Elaine Walker, PhD, served as collaborators. Chapter 2, What Are the Symptoms of Psychosis?, initially developed by Tandrea Carter, PhD, provides descriptions and explanations of the symptoms of psychosis. Philip Harvey, PhD, served as a collaborator for this chapter. In Chapter 3, What Diagnoses Are Associated with Psychosis?, we describe psychosis due to a medical condition, drug-induced psychosis, and a number of psychiatric diagnoses associated with psychosis. We also explain how mental health professionals decide on a certain diagnosis. Amy Leiner, PhD, assisted with initial chapter development, and Ross Norman, PhD, served as a collaborator. In Chapter 4, What Causes Psychotic Disorders Like Schizophrenia?, we describe the main models pertaining to causes and the different risk factors for developing psychosis. For this chapter, Kevin Tessner, PhD, assisted with initial development, and Matthew Broome, MRCPsych, PhD, served as a collaborator.

Part II, Clarifying the Initial Evaluation and Treatment of Psychosis, focuses on the evaluation process, medicines, psychosocial treatments used to treat psychosis, as well as the importance of sticking with treatment. In Chapter 5, The Initial Evaluation of Psychosis, we describe the thorough evaluation that a patient is given when beginning treatment. We explain in detail the interview, lab tests, and imaging tests that he or she may be given. For this chapter, Hanan Trotman, MA, assisted with initial development. Chapter 6, Medicines Used to Treat Psychosis, describes the categories of medicines used for psychosis, as well as the way they work in one's body. It also weighs the pros and cons of these types of medicines and describes the sometimes difficult process of finding the right medicine. In Chapter 7, Psychosocial Treatments for Early Psychosis, we explain the importance of psychosocial treatments as well as the multiple types of treatments that may be recommended. Hanan Trotman, MA, assisted with initial development, and Jean Addington, PhD, and Eóin Killackey, DPsych, served as collaborators. In Chapter 8, Follow-Up and Sticking with Treatment, we explain why it is important to stick with treatment and ways to encourage adherence. For this chapter, Erin Bergner, MPH, assisted with initial chapter writing, and Ashok Malla, MBBS, FRCPC, MRCPsch, and Srividya Iyer, PhD, served as collaborators.

Part III, Helping You Look Ahead to Next Steps, focuses on coping and recovery, as well as where and how to seek additional resources and information. Chapter 9, Early Warning Signs and Preventing a Relapse, describes early relapse symptoms that may come before another episode of psychosis. Sandra Goulding, MPH, assisted with initial chapter development, and Kristin Cadenhead, MD, served as a collaborator. In Chapter 10, Staying Healthy, we present some of the challenges faced by those beginning recovery and resources that may be helpful in overcoming these challenges. This chapter was initially developed by Michelle Esterberg, MPH, MA, and Brian Kirkpatrick, MD, MSPH, served as a collaborator. In Chapter 11, Promoting Recovery, we explain the new recovery movement in mental health and its basic principles. Michelle Esterberg, MPH, MA, assisted in writing the chapter, and Robert Drake, MD, PhD, and Jacqueline Feldman, MD, served as expert collaborators. In Chapter 12, Fighting Stigma, we explain the concept of stigma and how it affects people with psychosis and their families. We also provide ways that you can deal with stigma. Lauren Franz, MBChB, MPH, assisted with initial chapter development, and Amy Watson, PhD, served as a collaborator. Chapter 13, Reducing Stress, Coping, and Communicating Effectively: Tips for Family Members and Patients, provides information on how families can increase communication, reduce stress, and assist their loved ones with sticking with treatment. This chapter was initially developed with assistance from Sandra Goulding, MPH, and Nadine J. Kaslow, PhD, was a collaborator. In Chapter 14, Finding Specialized

Programs for Early Psychosis, we describe early psychosis clinical programs and provide information on individual programs from around the world. We also briefly describe prodromal clinics and provide information on these programs as well. Claire Ramsay, MPH, assisted with initial chapter development, and Jane Edwards, PhD, and Tor Larsen, MD, PhD, served as expert international collaborators. In Chapter 15, Seeking More Information, we explain the importance of educating yourself on psychosis and different ways to go about seeking this information. In our final chapter, Understanding Mental Health First Aid, we provide first aid guidelines developed by Betty Kitchener, BA, MNse, and Anthony Jorm, PhD, DSc. Their guidelines explain how to provide mental health "first aid" to those who may be experiencing an episode of psychosis.

We believe that recovery is possible. Life can be good again. We chose the image shown on the cover, drawn by a man in recovery himself, to represent this belief. We view the faces as representative of diversity, optimism, and the promise of recovery.

However, our optimism is balanced by a deep recognition of how serious the first episode of psychosis is. We strongly encourage patients and families to seek evaluation and treatment as soon as possible, to heed the advice of experienced mental health professionals, and to stick with treatment. We believe that through collaboration with experts in the treatment of psychosis, patients and their families have the best chance to move beyond psychosis towards recovery.

Michael T. Compton, MD, MPH, and Beth Broussard, MPH, CHES
Emory University School of Medicine, Department of Psychiatry and Behavioral Sciences, Atlanta, Georgia, United States

Table of Contents

List of Figures, Tables, and Worksheets

I   Answering Your Basic Questions

1   What Is Psychosis?

We began the Preface with a list of questions that people experiencing psychosis and their family members often have. As we mentioned, an episode of psychosis can be frightening, confusing, and painful for the individual going through it and for his or her family members. We also noted that this book is meant to help readers through a very difficult time by providing much needed information. Part 1 of this book, Answering Your Basic Questions, focuses on explaining some of the most important facts about psychosis. This chapter addresses the first basic question, what is psychosis?

In this chapter, we define what psychosis *is* and then dispel some myths by describing what psychosis is *not*. We then briefly describe what percentage of people develop psychosis and when it usually first begins. Next, we present the idea of a "psychosis continuum," which means that experiences of psychosis can differ in level of seriousness. We then set the stage for later chapters by briefly introducing schizo-phrenia (one of the illnesses that is related to psychosis) and several other topics to come later in the book, including causes of psychosis, treatments, and recovery.

What Psychosis Is

Psychosis is a form of mental illness. A **mental illness** affects a person's thoughts, feelings, and behaviors. Like physical illnesses, mental illnesses are treatable. Psychosis is a treatable mental illness syndrome. You may be familiar with some other mental illness syndromes, such as depression, posttraumatic stress disorder, and panic attacks.

So what exactly does psychosis mean? **Psychosis** is a word used to describe a person's mental state when he or she is out of touch with reality. For example, a person might hear voices that are not really there (auditory hallucinations) or believe things that are not really true (delusions). Psychosis is a medical condition that occurs due to a dysfunction in the brain. People with psychosis have difficulty separating false personal experiences from reality. They may behave in a bizarre or risky manner without realizing that they are doing anything unusual.

> Psychosis is a medical condition that occurs due to a dysfunction in the brain. People with psychosis have difficulty separating false, personal experiences from reality.

Similar to any other health condition, psychosis consists of a combination of both *symptoms* that patients experience and *signs* that doctors observe. This combination of symptoms and signs is a syndrome. All three of these terms—symptoms, signs, and syndrome—are described in detail in Chapter 2. Some of the many *symptoms* of psychosis may include hearing voices when there is really no one there and feeling overly frightened or paranoid. Some of the many *signs* of psychosis may include being withdrawn, having confused thoughts, or displaying odd behaviors. However, the difference between signs and symptoms is not always clear. Some "symptoms" experienced by the patient can also be seen as "signs" observed by others. We roughly divide illness features into signs and symptoms but admit that there is no real distinction in some cases.

A **psychotic episode** is a period of time during which someone has psychotic symptoms. These symptoms make it difficult for an individual to carry out daily activities. A psychotic episode may last from days to years. In some cases, psychotic-like symptoms may last for only minutes or hours. People who have a **psychotic disorder** have a mental illness that brings about psychosis which interferes with life. The various psychotic disorders and other disorders that may cause psychosis are described in detail in Chapter 3. Some people with a psychotic disorder have repeating episodes, but are able to function normally between these episodes. Others may experience only one psychotic episode in their lifetime.

An episode of psychosis can seriously disrupt one's functioning. Both "positive symptoms," such as hallucinations and delusions, and "negative symptoms," such as decreased energy and motivation, can interfere with school or work. (Again, these and other types of symptoms are described in detail in Chapter 2.) In more serious cases, such symptoms can lead to quitting school or to losing one's job.

Before a psychotic episode, family and friends may notice changes in emotions, behaviors, thinking, and beliefs about oneself and the world. For example, they may see changes in things such as mood, sleep habits, social activities, beliefs, or behaviors. These changes, often called **prodromal symptoms**, are some of the early warning signs for a psychotic illness (see Chapter 2 on What are the Symptoms of Psychosis? and Chapter 9 on Early Warning Signs and Preventing a Relapse).

The experience of psychosis is unique for each person who has it. For some people, problems with substance abuse, self-harm, or confusion may start or get worse with an episode of psychosis. Others may feel more tension or distrust while having a psychotic episode. Family and friends should know that any unexpected or aggressive behavior is likely a reaction to hallucinations and/or delusions, which are very real for the person with psychosis. It is important to realize that bizarre thoughts or behaviors are part of a treatable illness; family and friends should understand that their loved one often does not have control over these thoughts and behaviors. So, although the symptoms of psychosis may be frightening to the patient and his or her family, there are good treatments for these symptoms. Friends and family members should try to help the individual to receive the right mental health treatment.

First-episode psychosis is simply the period of time when a person first begins to experience psychosis. This book focuses on the first episode of psychosis because it is during this time that patients and families need detailed information about the initial evaluation and treatment. Some researchers think of the first five years during and after a first episode of psychosis as a **critical period**. That is, the early phase of psychosis is very important because it is during this time that long-term outcome may be most improved by treatment. This is also a critical period because crucial psychological and social skills are developing, and mental health professionals want to minimize the damage to these skills that psychosis can cause. It is vital that patients and families receive help in order to reduce symptoms and promote recovery. Researchers believe that the first psychotic episode and the critical period deserve special, thorough, and ongoing treatment in order to provide patients the best possible outcomes.

What Psychosis is NOT

Before learning more about psychosis, it is important to address some common myths about psychosis.

- **Psychosis is not multiple personality disorder.** In multiple personality disorder (a very rare psychiatric disorder), a person unconsciously has two or more separate personalities. Each personality has its own thoughts, feelings, and behaviors. Although people with psychosis may hear other voices or behave in response to delusions, they do not alternate between different personalities. So, psychosis is not "split personality" or multiple personality disorder.

- **Psychosis is not insanity.** The word *insanity* is a legal term often meaning that one is too mentally ill to be held responsible for a crime (as in the phrase "not guilty by reason of insanity"). A very small percentage of individuals with psychosis fall into this legal classification. Usually, people with psychosis are not legally insane, nor do they usually commit crimes. Insanity is a word that is no longer used in the medical field.

- **People with psychosis are not simply "crazy."** The word *psychotic* describes someone who is experiencing the condition of psychosis. Society has wrongly used the word psychotic to describe someone who is "crazy" or out of control. People with psychosis should not be called crazy; instead, they are suffering from a treatable mental illness. Mental health professionals view the word *crazy* as an outdated and damaging word, like *insanity* or *lunacy*. Nowadays, medical professionals try to avoid the word *crazy* because it leads to stigma (see Chapter 12). So, even though it is a commonly used word in society, referring to someone as "crazy" is hurtful.

- **Psychosis is not psychopathy.** Psychopathy is a personality disorder in which people lack sympathy, have no regret for criminal or violent behaviors, and are socially manipulative. Although both mental illnesses contain the prefix *psycho*, they are very different in nature. Most people diagnosed with psychosis are not violent, and most people diagnosed with psychopathy (also called sociopathy or antisocial personality disorder) do not have hallucinations or delusions. So, psychosis does not equal psychopathy or criminal behavior.

- **Psychosis is not delirium.** People with delirium, or a state of confusion, may have trouble with memory and concentration. They may be disoriented, meaning that they do not know the date, where they are, or possibly even who they are (see Chapter 3 on What Are the Different Diagnoses Related to Psychosis?). Although some people with psychosis have poor memory, they generally know who they are, where they are, and what the date is. So, psychosis is not the same as being delirious. Psychosis is also very different from dementia, which is a slowly developing state of confusion that usually occurs in the elderly (see Chapter 3).

- **People with psychosis are usually not a threat to others.** In fact, they are at greater risk for injuring themselves than injuring others. Family and friends should understand that people with psychosis are rarely violent. They are suffering from an illness and need the same caring attention as people with diabetes, depression, or any other health condition.

- **People with psychosis are not completely disabled.** The experience of psychosis is different for every person who has it. Psychosis is more disabling for some people than for others because of individual differences in personality, social support, genes, and experiences. The right treatment can help lessen or remove the distressing symptoms of the illness. Many people with psychosis can recover to participate in their communities.

The word *psychotic* describes someone who is experiencing the condition of psychosis. Society has wrongly used the word psychotic to describe someone who is "crazy" or out of control. People with psychosis should not be called crazy; instead, they are suffering from a treatable mental illness.

Developing Psychosis

Very few people (about 3%, or 3 in 100) will experience an episode of psychosis in their lifetime. Psychosis affects both men and women across all cultures. Psychosis can happen at any time in life, but the onset or beginning of psychosis is usually in late adolescence or early adulthood. For men, the usual **age of onset** may be slightly earlier than for women. On average, men who develop a psychotic disorder experience their first psychotic symptoms up to three to five years before women do. For example, as described in Chapter 3, the symptoms of schizophrenia usually first become apparent in men between the ages of 20 and 30, and in women between the ages of 24 and 34. Schizophrenia is one of the most serious psychotic disorders, and about 1% of people will develop schizophrenia during the course of their lifetime (see Chapter 3).

The Psychosis Continuum

Everyone has some tendency to experience psychotic-like experiences or even psychosis, just as everyone has the potential to become depressed or anxious. *Normal* experiences that are similar to psychosis, though much milder, do not interfere with an individual's regular functioning. *Abnormal* experiences of psychosis interfere with functioning and make it difficult or impossible for a person to live a regular life. The more an experience interferes with daily life, the more serious the condition.

Researchers who study psychosis use the phrase **psychosis continuum** to describe the different levels of psychotic experiences. This simply means that there is a range of **severity** or seriousness across the different types of experiences of psychosis. The different types of psychotic experiences range from normal experiences that are similar to psychosis and that cause little or no distress, to the full syndrome of psychosis that causes a lot of distress or problems in life. Although normal, psychotic-like experiences are fairly common, psychotic disorders that cause the full syndrome of psychosis are quite rare. Figure 1.1 illustrates how the different types of psychotic experiences relate to one another.

Some normal human experiences that do not affect regular functioning are similar to psychosis. They cause no distress and do not interfere with life. We have all had the occasional experience of wondering if someone might be talking about us (which is a normal curiosity) or thinking that we hear the phone ring while taking a shower (which is a normal experience of attention being drawn to sounds that may be heard over noise).

Some people occasionally may have minor psychotic-like symptoms, such as hearing a voice or suspecting that someone is following them. These brief, infrequent symptoms do not disrupt functioning. About one-fourth (25%, or 25 out of 100) of the general population experiences these types of symptoms in their lifetime. These are brief psychotic experiences that usually go away, not the full syndrome of psychosis. Psychosis is an exaggeration of these experiences—to the point that they become troubling and interfere with life—caused by a dysfunction in the brain.

Certain experiences can cause a psychotic episode, such as major stress, drug use, and even some medical problems. Some examples of psychosis caused by stressors include **stress-induced psychosis**, **drug-induced psychosis**, and **psychosis related to a medical problem**. People who experience a great deal of physical stress from lack of sleep, hunger, or torture may experience stress-induced psychosis. Drug-induced psychosis may happen when a person is using drugs like cocaine, LSD, marijuana, methamphetamine, or PCP. People with certain physical illnesses, such as meningitis, seizures, or a brain tumor, may experience psychosis related to a medical problem (see Chapter 3). In all of these cases, the symptoms of psychosis often, but not always, go away after removing the stressor, drug, or medical problem. Some people do not fully recover from an episode of psychosis if the stressor

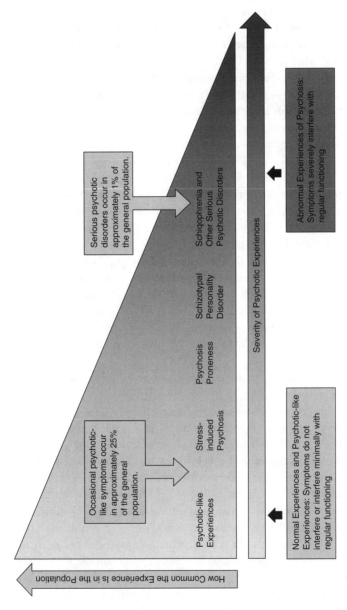

Figure 1.1 The Psychosis Continuum. Shown here is the range of severity among the different types of psychotic-like and full psychotic experiences. These experiences range from normal experiences that produce no or minimal levels of distress (left side) to abnormal experiences that cause a lot of distress (right side).

or cause of psychosis is too intense or lasts for too long, or if they are at risk for a psychotic illness.

Some people are particularly at risk for psychosis due to their genes or due to exposure to "environmental" factors that may have occurred in early life. Such factors may include having an infection as a fetus or baby, a difficult labor or delivery when being born, or having had a head injury (see Chapter 4 on What Causes Primary Psychotic Disorders Like Schizophrenia?). It should be noted that having any one or more of these risk factors increases one's risk only slightly.

Some people are more likely to develop psychotic symptoms than others. That is, some people are more **psychosis-prone** than others. They may or may not develop psychosis. People who experience mild, ongoing difficulties from symptoms but can still function well enough to work and maintain relationships may have **schizotypal personality features**. People with schizotypal personality styles can seem to have fewer social skills at times because of suspicious or paranoid thinking. They also tend to withdraw from society. Typically, they do not experience full hallucinations or delusions, and they can manage to live independently. When many schizotypal personality features are present and long-lasting, a person might be diagnosed by mental health professionals as having **schizotypal personality disorder**. Schizotypal personality disorder is a stable set of personality traits that appear as a milder form of the symptoms of schizophrenia.

People who have a full syndrome of psychosis usually have serious problems in life. They may be unable to work, attend school, or participate in some social activities. Either hallucinations, delusions, or both may be present. In addition, people with psychosis may experience slow or confused thinking and speech, and their behavior may be odd or risky. People with this experience of psychosis may have schizophrenia or another serious primary psychotic disorder. On the other hand, they may have a different type of mental illness, such as depression with psychotic features or bipolar disorder (also called manic-depressive illness). We describe these different psychiatric illnesses that can cause psychosis in more detail in Chapter 3.

> People who have a full syndrome of psychosis usually have serious problems in life. They may be unable to work, attend school, or participate in some social activities.

There are also cases when the cause of a psychotic-like experience is not as clear. For example, some people have reported abilities related to their spirituality or religion, such as seeing or hearing things that other people cannot. These experiences usually do not interfere with an individual's functioning, and one's specific religion or culture considers them to be normal or special experiences. This book focuses on the types of psychotic experiences that are abnormal or disabling.

Schizophrenia and Other Serious Psychotic Disorders

When someone has a headache, he or she may not know what is causing the headache. Is the headache from stress? Does the person have a cold or the flu? Or is the headache related to something more serious, like high blood pressure, or even a brain tumor? If the headache worsens or does not go away, it is a good idea to visit the doctor for medical evaluation and treatment. In the same way, psychosis can happen in several different illnesses, mostly in mental disorders. For example, people with severe depression, bipolar disorder, or schizophrenia can have a psychotic episode. There are many different types of psychotic disorders, and all are recognizable by the types of symptoms and how long those symptoms last.

For example, schizophrenia is a type of psychotic disorder in which at least two of the following occur for at least one month, but often much longer: hallucinations, delusions, disorganized speech, disorganized behavior, or "negative symptoms" (these symptoms are described in Chapter 2). Young people with a first-episode of psychosis may or may not go on to develop schizophrenia. Nevertheless, mental health professionals always recommend a thorough evaluation (see Chapter 5 on The Initial Evaluation of Psychosis), treatment (see Chapters 6 on Medicines Used to Treat Psychosis and 7 on Psychosocial Treatments for Early Psychosis) and follow-up (see Chapter 8 on Follow-up and Sticking with Treatment).

Schizophrenia is only one type of psychotic disorder, as described in Chapter 3. Others include schizophreniform disorder, schizoaffective disorder, and psychotic disorder not otherwise specified. These disorders differ from schizophrenia by the types of symptoms involved and the length of time those symptoms last.

In fact, all mental illnesses are defined by a specific group or set of symptoms. For example, people with obsessive-compulsive disorder do not hallucinate, but people with psychosis often do. In other words, the symptoms of obsessive-compulsive disorder, depression, social anxiety disorder, autism, or a number of other mental disorders differ from the symptoms of psychosis. Psychotic disorders have a unique set of symptoms that make them different from other mental illnesses, placing them in their own class of disorders.

Possible Causes of Psychosis

Although Chapter 4 goes into detail about the causes of psychosis, it is important to begin to understand the causes here. People who study psychosis believe there are two main models for the causes of the illness. These two models are not competing; they go hand in hand. One involves the developing brain (**neurodevelopmental model**), and the other is about the relationship between genes and stress (**diathesis-stress model**).

Psychosis is a medical condition of the brain, but scientists have not figured out exactly what is happening in the brain to cause this illness. Some think that it is a result of minor injuries to the brain during its growth and development. They call this idea the neurodevelopmental model. Injuries to the brain can happen for several reasons. For example, brain injuries can happen if a pregnant mother uses harmful drugs or if some physical trauma happens while the fetal brain is developing.

Adolescence is a time when the brain goes through some major changes. The minor brain injuries that may have happened during fetal brain development may become more apparent in adolescence when the brain develops further. These injuries can start to affect a person's thinking, feelings, and behavior. That is, some doctors think that psychosis happens as an individual is maturing in adolescence because he or she was born with minor injuries to the brain. This view explains why psychotic illnesses rarely occur in young children. Additionally, it can explain why first-episode psychosis is most common in late adolescence and young adulthood.

The other main explanation for why psychosis happens involves the relationship between genes and the environment one lives in. In this diathesis-stress model, some people are born with genes that put them at greater risk for having psychosis. However, genes alone are not enough to start a psychotic episode. There must be a stressor to trigger an episode, such as a major life event or extended drug use. The combination of certain genes and a stressor can cause psychosis. For people who are psychosis-prone due to certain genes or early life environmental risk factors, a crisis, stressful life event, or drug of abuse could cause the onset of psychosis. Again, Chapter 4 provides much more detail on the causes of psychotic disorders like schizophrenia.

Taking Action: Treatment and Recovery

There are three phases of psychosis. The first is the **prodromal phase**, the time before a psychotic episode when warning signs first appear. The prodromal phase may last from several weeks to several years. The **acute phase** is the time during the psychotic episode when symptoms are most disruptive. The acute phase usually lasts until treatment is sought and symptoms are first evaluated and treated. The third is the **recovery phase** or the time after the psychotic episode when symptoms of psychosis lessen or sometimes go away completely with treatment. The recovery phase is often considered to be the first 6–18 months of treatment.

People who get treatment in the earlier stages of the illness often do better than people who wait a long time before getting treatment. However, recognizing psychosis in its early stages can be challenging. Some symptoms, such as mood changes or sleep disturbances, can easily be confused with normal changes of adolescence (see Chapter 9 on Early Warning Signs and Preventing a Relapse).

The best help for someone with psychosis is to be active about seeking treatment and following through completely with treatment. To be active about seeking treatment means doing several things. It means going to the doctor as soon as any disturbing symptoms appear. It also means learning about psychosis by talking to others or reading books. There are many resources in the community, as well as on the Internet, to help understand this experience (see Chapter 15 on Seeking More Information). When visiting the doctor, do not hesitate to ask questions or express concerns. Psychosis is a serious, but treatable, mental illness.

A psychotic episode can be a frightening and stressful experience for both the person with psychosis and his or her loved ones. Untreated psychosis can disrupt the life of both the individual and his or her family and friends. It is perfectly understandable that both the person and his or her family members would feel scared, disappointed, or upset when dealing with the new onset of psychotic symptoms. However, these normal feelings should not interfere with seeking treatment. Psychosis, though often frightening and confusing, should be treated promptly when at all possible, like any other illness.

For the majority of individuals with first-episode psychosis, their "positive" psychotic symptoms (such as hallucinations or delusions) will clear up partially or completely within weeks of starting treatment. Treatment includes both medicine (see Chapter 6) and psychosocial interventions (see Chapter 7). Hospitalization is sometimes needed. Following through with treatment is necessary to recover. Recovery, which is much broader than just eliminating symptoms, is described in detail in Chapter 11.

Putting It All Together

Psychosis is a treatable disorder of the brain that disrupts an individual's ability to understand the difference between personal experiences and reality. Many of society's ideas about psychosis are not true, such as the notion that people with psychosis have multiple personality disorder, are insane, are dangerous, or are completely disabled. Everyone has the potential to experience some psychotic-like experiences or even psychosis. The continuum of psychosis ranges from normal, everyday experiences that interfere very little in people's lives to more serious experiences that greatly interfere with everyday life. The many different types of psychotic disorders differ in the types and duration of symptoms associated with them. We explain these symptoms and diagnoses in Chapters 2 and 3.

While the exact cause of psychosis is not yet known, there are two main hypotheses. One is the neurodevelopmental hypothesis, which means that psychosis is a result of minor injuries to the brain during its growth and development. The second is the diathesis-stress model, which means that psychosis is a result of the relationship between genes and the environment one lives in.

> People who get treatment in the earlier stages of the illness do better than people who wait a long time before getting treatment.

Even though researchers are still trying to figure out the exact causes of psychosis, effective treatments are available. For most people with psychosis, many symptoms clear up with treatment, and they can move forward with their life goals through recovery. It is important to actively seek treatment and stick with it. This will help to increase chances of recovery and reduce relapse and rehospitalization.

Key Chapter Points

- ☛ Psychosis is a medical condition that occurs due to a dysfunction in the brain.
- ☛ Only a small percentage of people (about 3%) will experience an episode of psychosis at some time in their life. Even fewer (about 1%) will develop schizophrenia, one of the psychotic disorders.
- ☛ The onset of psychosis is usually in late adolescence or early adulthood.
- ☛ The causes of psychosis are related to the developing brain and an interaction between genes and the environment.
- ☛ People who get treatment in the earlier stages of the illness often do better than people who delay getting treatment.
- ☛ For most people with first-episode psychosis, psychotic symptoms clear up partially or completely within weeks of starting treatment.
- ☛ Being active about seeking treatment and following through with treatment is important for moving towards recovery.

Acknowledgments: This chapter was originally developed and written by Victoria H. Chien, BA, and Michelle L. Esterberg, MPH, MA. Cheryl Corcoran, MD, and Elaine F. Walker, PhD, served as collaborators for this chapter.

2 What Are the Symptoms of Psychosis?

Before learning about the symptoms of psychosis, it is important to understand what doctors mean by the words *symptoms*, *signs*, *syndromes*, and *diagnosis*. In this chapter, we explain these four words and then describe the various symptoms of early psychosis.

Nearly any illness, whether it affects the body or the brain, causes **symptoms**. A symptom is an obvious change from one's normal health that happens when an illness or disease occurs. For example, symptoms of a heart attack may include chest pain, pressure in the chest, pain running down the left arm, problems breathing, nausea, and sweating. Symptoms of the flu may include fever, chills, cough, sore throat, and nausea. Symptoms often are the reason you go to a doctor or other health-care provider. The doctor then examines the patient to look for **signs**. Signs are like symptoms, but a doctor sees them through an interview, exam, or test, while symptoms are experienced by the patient. The patient may not even know that he or she has signs of an illness. For example, during a routine check-up, the doctor may discover that the patient has high blood pressure or high cholesterol. These signs could mean that the patient has heart disease or is at risk for a heart attack.

Most medical diseases and mental illnesses cause both symptoms that patients experience and signs that doctors observe. A combination of both symptoms and signs is a **syndrome**. A heart attack is an example of a medical syndrome. Another example, diabetes, has symptoms such as being thirsty and frequent urination, and signs such as high levels of glucose, or sugar, in the blood. Some other medical syndromes are an ear infection, the flu, arthritis, and stroke. There also are many types of mental illness syndromes, such as depression, panic attacks, psychosis, and dementia. This book focuses on the syndrome of psychosis (see Chapter 1). It especially focuses on the first time psychosis appears, usually between the ages of 16 and 30 years.

The word **diagnosis** (plural, **diagnoses**) refers to the specific medical word(s) given to an illness or syndrome by health-care providers. Examples of medical diagnoses include "diabetes mellitus" (diabetes), "acute myocardial infarction" (heart attack), and "cerebrovascular accident" (stroke). Diagnoses of mental illnesses include "bipolar disorder," "major depressive disorder," and "Alzheimer's disease." As discussed in Chapter 3, diagnoses of "schizophrenia," "schizophreniform disorder," "schizoaffective disorder," and other related psychiatric illnesses form a category of illnesses called primary psychotic disorders, because they all cause psychosis.

Like many other mental illnesses, early psychosis is a syndrome that causes many different symptoms. People experiencing early psychosis have different types of symptoms, and one person's symptoms may change during the course of his or her illness. These many symptoms can be divided into several groups of symptoms. In this chapter, you will learn about nine groups of symptoms that may happen during early psychosis. The first three, positive symptoms, negative symptoms, and disorganized symptoms, are thought by some to be the three main groups of symptoms in psychotic disorders like schizophrenia. However, there are several other groups of symptoms that also may lead to problems, including impaired insight, cognitive dysfunction, hostile/aggressive symptoms, catatonic and movement symptoms, mood symptoms and anxiety, and suicidal thoughts.

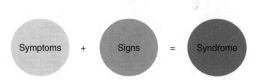

Figure 2.1 The Combination of Symptoms and Signs Is Called a Syndrome

People experiencing early psychosis have different types of symptoms, and one person's symptoms may change over the course of his or her illness.

We also discuss prodromal symptoms at the end of this chapter. Prodromal symptoms actually happen *before* psychosis begins. If you or someone you know has had an episode of psychosis, you may recall some of these slight symptoms that appeared before the psychotic symptoms began. These are important to learn about even though they happened in the past. A period of prodromal symptoms often happens before a future **relapse** or another episode of psychosis.

Positive Symptoms

The most outwardly obvious symptoms of psychosis are **positive symptoms**. The use of the word "positive" is often confusing and does not mean that these symptoms are enjoyable or helpful. They

Positive Symptoms	•Abnormal experiences *added on* to normal mental functions, such as hallucinations and delusions.
Negative Symptoms	•The *absence of* normal experiences, such as low motivation or loss of pleasure in hobbies.
Disorganized Symptoms	•The flow of thinking and speaking becomes out of order, confused, or jumbled.
Impaired Insight	•A lack of understanding of the symptoms or illness.
Cognitive Dysfunction	•Having problems with the process of thinking or with attention, learning, or memory.
Hostile/Aggressive Symptoms	•Having increased hostility or aggressivenss, often acting out of fear.
Catatonic/Movement Symptoms	•Problems with normal body movement that happen without a clear reason, such as appearing frozen.
Mood Symptoms and Anxiety	•Changes in one's moods or feelings and/or an increase in anxiety.
Suicidal Thoughts	•Thoughts about dying, wishing to be dead, or plans to commit suicide.

Figure 2.2 Nine Types of Symptoms of Early Psychosis

are things that people should not normally do or think. In other words, these symptoms are abnormal experiences *added on* to normal mental functions. Positive symptoms include hallucinations, delusions, suspiciousness/paranoia, and ideas of reference. Each of these is discussed in the pages that follow.

- **Hallucinations:** A hallucination is a false experience of one of the five senses (hearing, seeing, feeling, smelling, and tasting). Even though hallucinations may happen in any of the five senses, **auditory hallucinations** are the most common. Auditory hallucinations occur when someone hears voices, even though no one is really there speaking. These hallucinations may be voices calling one's name, commenting on one's actions, making harsh comments, or giving commands. Individuals with psychosis may react through behaviors—such as talking to oneself, whispering to oneself, or looking around as if someone else is talking—in response to the voices they are hearing. The voices are not made-up or imagined; the person who hears them is actually hearing the voice because of an abnormality in the brain. It is important to realize that the experience is very real to those who are hallucinating. Like other symptoms of psychosis, hallucinations are caused by a dysfunction in the brain.

- **Delusions:** A delusion is a false belief that lasts for a long period of time. There are several different types of delusions.
  - A **paranoid delusion** is the false belief that one is being plotted against or followed. For example, a person may believe that the FBI has planted a camera in the walls and his or her family is part of a government plot.
  - A **grandiose delusion** is the false belief that one has high social status, is famous, has large amounts of money, or has special powers.
  - A **religious delusion** is the false belief that one has religious importance, such as being a biblical figure.
  - A **somatic delusion** is the false belief that something is wrong with one's body. For example, a person may believe that there is a parasite in his or her skin or that a cancer or tumor is growing in his or her body.

° A **delusion of control** is the false belief that some other person or an outside force controls one's thoughts, feelings, or actions. For example, a person may be convinced that someone else is putting thoughts into his or her mind through a hex, a curse, or some other means.

Mental health professionals refer to delusions as *bizarre* when they are clearly impossible. For example, the belief that a remote control is influencing one's sense of smell is an example of a bizarre delusion. It is important to note that delusions are not just ideas or passing thoughts, they are firmly held beliefs. Even though some psychosocial interventions, like cognitive-behavioral therapy (see Chapter 7) may address the validity of delusions, it is usually not helpful to try to "talk someone out of his or her delusions" or try to prove the person wrong.

More than one positive symptom may occur at once. This state of being "out of touch with reality" is referred to as psychosis. The word psychotic means that someone is experiencing the condition of psychosis. For example, a person might hear voices that are not really there and believe things that are not really true. There are other symptoms that are related to positive symptoms that may be less severe in many cases and they are described next.

- **Suspiciousness/paranoia:** People with psychosis may experience suspiciousness when they feel that they cannot trust others. They may have an unexplained feeling that those around them are trying to cause problems in their life. Some suspicions may be so extreme that they form a paranoid delusion as described earlier. Other suspicions may be milder and result in people isolating themselves from others because they do not trust them. People with paranoia may not ask for help because they believe that others are trying to harm them.
- **Ideas of reference:** Ideas of reference happen when patients believe that people are talking about them or that things are referring especially to them when they really are not. For example, someone might believe that the television or radio newscasters are talking about him or her or are trying to send coded messages. This might prompt the person to remove or even destroy the television or radio because of these troubling false ideas.

Negative Symptoms

Another group of symptoms related to psychosis are the so-called **negative symptoms**. Negative symptoms are things that people should normally do or think but are now missing. In other words, these symptoms have *subtracted,* or removed, something from their experience, which is why they are called *negative symptoms.* Some negative symptoms described below include anhedonia; apathy; blunted affect or flat affect; emotional withdrawal; low drive, energy, or motivation; poor attention to grooming and hygiene; slow or empty thinking and speech; slow movements; and social isolation.

- **Anhedonia:** Anhedonia is a loss of interest or pleasure. People experiencing this symptom may not be able to find pleasure in experiences that they used to enjoy. They also may find that they are unable to fully enjoy fun and pleasant things like going to the movies, enjoying a tasty meal, or taking part in hobbies.
- **Apathy:** People with apathy tend not to care as deeply about what happens in their life. This may include not being upset about negative life events such as losing a job or failing in school.
- **Blunted affect:** People with blunted affect show less outward emotion than normal. This is observed as decreased facial expression, less use of body language, and a dull tone of voice. A **flat affect** is an extreme lessening of outward emotion, worse than blunted affect. People with a flat affect have an almost complete absence of facial expressions and body language, resulting in a very dull appearance and tone of voice.
- **Emotional withdrawal:** People with emotional withdrawal lack emotional closeness to others. They do not feel like they belong or connect with others, even when spending time with other people.
- **Low drive, energy, or motivation:** People experiencing this symptom may have lost the desire to finish school, be in a relationship, get a job, or engage in social activities.
- **Poor attention to grooming and hygiene:** Poor attention to grooming and hygiene can include not bathing, not brushing one's teeth, wearing dirty clothes, or not combing one's hair. This neglect can happen for many reasons, including a lower ability to care for oneself and a decreased understanding of how to act in social situations. It may also be the result of apathy and low motivation.

- **Slow or empty thinking and speech:** People experiencing this symptom may seem like they are unable to keep up with the conversation. There may also be a long period between asking a question and their response to it. It may seem like they have very few thoughts or a limited range of thoughts.
- **Slow movements:** Individuals with slow movements as a negative symptom may walk, move, and talk much more slowly than normal.
- **Social isolation:** People experiencing social isolation may become unconcerned with relationships that had been close and important to them before. They usually have difficulty forming new relationships. They may instead spend most of their time alone.

While these negative symptoms are less obvious than positive symptoms, they can have an equally adverse impact on someone by making it very hard to attend school, keep a job, and have relationships. People should not mistake negative symptoms for laziness or an attitude problem. This wrongly blames the patient for serious symptoms that are not under his or her control.

Although positive symptoms tend to vary between better and worse over time, negative symptoms are often longer-lasting. Unfortunately, the medicines currently available are less effective at treating negative symptoms than positive symptoms (see Chapter 6 on Medicines Used to Treat Psychosis).

Psychosis is a medical condition that occurs due to a dysfunction in the brain. People with psychosis have difficulty separating false, personal experience from reality.

Disorganized Symptoms

Often in psychosis, there are signs of **disorganization** of thoughts and speech. The normal flow of thinking and speaking can become out of order, confusing, and jumbled. Two examples of disorganization of thoughts are derailment and loosening of associations.

- **Derailment:** Derailment happens when one idea connects to the next, but the thoughts become confusing because they go off on a tangent and end on a different subject. Derailment might sound like this: "I'm hungry. I need to go to the store to get a loaf of bread because bread is the staff of life. The staff members at my college seem too busy. They need more help..." Here, the patient starts talking about one topic, but veers off on an unrelated tangent and never gets back to the original topic. The original thought becomes derailed along the way.

- **Loosening of associations:** Unlike derailment, loosening of association is when one idea does not match the next at all. The ideas do not connect in any logical way. It might sound like this: "I go to the chair and a balloon is seen because of the traffic signal." Ideas shift from one subject to another in a completely unrelated way. The thinking process is "loose" instead of being tightly ordered and reasonable.

In both derailment and loosening of associations, the disorganized thoughts come across as confused and confusing. Other problems with the ability to think clearly include poverty of content of speech and thought blocking.

- **Poverty of content of speech:** This means that what one is talking about may appear unclear, meaningless, or vague. For example, a person may have the same answer for every question asked, or have very, very little to say. This is very similar to the negative symptom of slow or empty thinking and speech.
- **Thought blocking:** Thought blocking happens when there is an interruption in the train of thought and the person cannot put his or her thoughts into words. The thoughts are "blocked" from coming out. Thus, the person may be very slow to respond to questions or may not be able to respond at all.

In addition to these types of disorganized thoughts, patients may also have **disorganized behavior**. Disorganized behavior often appears as an inability to follow through with plans. It may also be seen in a bizarre appearance, such as having shoes on the wrong feet or wearing clothes inside out. People may dress inappropriately for the weather, wearing several layers of clothing even in warm temperatures. Thus, behavior may become disorganized, usually because one's thoughts are disorganized.

Impaired Insight

Unfortunately, **impaired insight** (often referred to as "unawareness of illness") is a common problem for people with psychosis. Impaired insight occurs when those experiencing psychotic symptoms are not fully aware of their behavior or the condition of their mind. Because their unusual experiences may be very real to them, they do not realize that the thoughts and behaviors they are having are a change from their normal self. They also may be unaware that their behavior is socially unacceptable and different from that of other people. Impaired insight is surely one of the most difficult problems to deal with in the syndrome of psychosis, especially for health-care providers and family members who desperately want patients to understand the illness and realize the benefits of treatment. People with impaired insight often refuse to take medicines or follow up with treatment. Health-care providers try to teach people with psychosis more about their symptoms so that their insight will improve. This helps patients to adhere to, or stick with, their treatment (see Chapter 8 on Follow-up and Sticking with Treatment) and leads to better results for their illness.

> Impaired insight occurs when those experiencing psychotic symptoms are not fully aware of their behavior or the condition of their mind. Because their unusual experiences may be very real to them, they do not realize that the thoughts and behaviors they are having are a change from their normal self.

Cognitive Dysfunction

The term **cognitive dysfunction** refers to symptoms that cause problems with some of the most important mental functions, like concentration, learning, memory, and planning. Although people with psychosis typically have a close to normal intelligence or IQ (intelligence quotient), they may have some problems with specific cognitive abilities, like the ability to understand, process, and recall information. Everyone has problems remembering things or paying attention sometimes. However, people with psychosis have more severe problems that last for a longer period of time.

The forms of cognitive dysfunction that are part of psychosis may include difficulties with abstract thinking, poor attention and concentration, impaired information processing, language problems, poor memory, and difficulties with planning. These frequently go along with negative symptoms. Even though cognitive dysfunction often goes unnoticed, it can cause major problems at school or on the job. Cognitive dysfunction tends to be somewhat long-lasting over time, mostly silent, and easy to overlook, but very problematic. Doctors assess for cognitive dysfunction using a group of **cognitive tests**, also referred to as neurocognitive tests, neuropsychological tests, or psychological tests.

- **Difficulties with abstract thinking:** People with psychosis may not be able to understand complex concepts or solve problems that require them to think through several steps. In addition, they may find it difficult to understand ideas with abstract meanings, such as proverbs or sayings. For example, they may not understand common phrases, like "don't put all your eggs in one basket," "don't judge a book by its cover," or "there's no use crying over spilled milk."
- **Poor attention and concentration:** People experiencing psychosis often display limited attention and concentration. They may have a hard time keeping their thoughts on one idea. They also may find tasks that require them to focus their attention very tiring. For example, they may find it difficult to stay focused on a book or a television show for more than a few minutes.
- **Impaired information processing:** People experiencing this symptom may have difficulty sorting out information and discovering meaning in things that they observe. It may appear that things do not "sink in" the way they used to or that complex things seem more difficult for them to understand than before.
- **Language problems:** People with psychosis may have trouble writing or speaking. Language problems also may include using words incorrectly, using new words that do not really have a recognized meaning, or using words because of what they sound like rather than because of their meanings.

- **Poor memory:** People experiencing poor memory usually have trouble learning and remembering new things. Some also may have trouble remembering past events, but this is less common.
- **Difficulties with planning:** Cognitive dysfunction that occurs with psychosis may make it hard to plan. People may have trouble focusing on future events in a logical way. They also may not have the ability to correctly judge different plans of action. In addition, they may become uncertain and have difficulty committing to one plan.

Hostile/Aggressive Symptoms

Most people experiencing psychosis are not dangerous or violent in any way, and the rate of violence in people experiencing psychosis is very similar to that of the population as a whole. However, some people with psychosis do show increased **hostility** or **aggressiveness**. They may argue more than normal, destroy property, or make threats towards others. Although rare, when these behaviors do occur, they can be driven by specific delusions. For example, someone with a paranoid delusion may act out of fear, believing that he or she must do something for protection and safety.

Catatonic and Movement Symptoms

Catatonia is a rare syndrome that can happen together with the syndrome of psychosis. It is a severe change from normal body movements that happens without a clear reason. For example, those who have catatonia may lose the ability to move, appearing frozen, stiff, and motionless. They also may appear completely unresponsive to their environment. People with psychosis may experience less extreme movement symptoms including a very slow rate of movement as well as unnatural motions or poses. Catatonia can be dangerous because it can keep people from getting adequate nutrition, from taking care of their hygiene, and from taking medicine. In some instances, it can also cause a dangerous elevation in vital signs, such as blood pressure.

Sometimes antipsychotic medicines, especially the older "conventional" medicines, may cause movement side effects that mimic the symptoms of catatonia. But, in this case, the movement side effects (like slowness, stiffness, or tremor) are an unwanted effect of the medicines. Catatonia, on the other hand, consists of movement signs and symptoms not caused by medicine, but by the illness itself.

Mood Symptoms and Anxiety

Although some people with a psychotic disorder may experience or express emotions less deeply, as described earlier (anhedonia, apathy, or blunted or flat affect); for others, psychosis can cause other types of changes in their mood. Some of these mood symptoms may be like the ones seen in other mental illnesses, like major depression or bipolar disorder. So, it is possible that some people with psychosis may have prominent negative symptoms and a decreased expression of emotions. However, others may have few or no negative symptoms but have some symptoms commonly seen in depression. Yet others may have some of the mood symptoms often seen in **mania**, the syndrome that occurs in people with bipolar disorder (also called manic-depressive illness).

Changes in one's moods or feelings may come before psychosis, occur during a first episode of psychosis, or come after a psychotic episode. For instance, some people may experience a **depressed mood**, or **depression**. They may feel down, unhappy, or empty.

On the other hand, people with psychosis also may experience a syndrome called mania, or periods in which they feel abnormally happy, high, energetic, or excited. An exaggerated sense of self-worth, belief that one has special powers, and reckless or dangerous behaviors may also be seen in mania. Some people have a **labile affect** in which their mood quickly moves between happy and sad, such as laughing that quickly switches to crying. When someone repeatedly smiles or laughs out of context, this is called an **inappropriate affect.**

It is also common for people experiencing psychosis to be anxious or nervous. One source of **anxiety** may be delusional thoughts. For example, a patient may think that people are following him or her and plotting murder. Anxiety may show up in some people as being tense or jittery, worrying that something bad is going to happen, or appearing generally uneasy in most situations.

Suicidal Thoughts

People experiencing psychosis may have thoughts about dying. This may include wishing to be dead, as well as thinking about or planning to commit suicide. **Suicidal thoughts** may be driven by several symptoms, including emotional distress due to the frightening experience of psychosis or as a direct result of hallucinations or delusions. For example, a person may hear voices instructing him or her to commit suicide.

In addition, people who have some level of insight into how they have changed may become hopeless and depressed. Suicidal thoughts may also happen if patients become aware that they may not be able to achieve goals as they had planned. People with psychosis are at a much higher risk for suicide attempts and completed suicide than the population as a whole. Family and friends should, therefore, take any expression of suicidal thoughts very seriously.

> People who have some level of insight into how they have changed may become hopeless and depressed. Suicidal thoughts may also happen if patients become aware that they may not be able to achieve goals as they had planned. People with psychosis are at a higher risk for suicide attempts and completed suicide. Family and friends should take any expression of suicidal thoughts very seriously.

Prodromal Symptoms

When mental health professionals speak of **prodromal symptoms,** they are talking about subtle changes in thoughts, feelings, or behaviors that happened *before* the first episode of psychosis. The prodromal period may last from a few days to a few years. Some people with psychosis may not have had any prodromal symptoms at all.

Prodromal symptoms are often similar to psychotic symptoms, just in a milder form. For example, a person may be very suspicious but not to the extent of having paranoid delusions. A person may mistake one object for another such as seeing spots on a wall as crawling bugs. Although this is a mistake, it is not a full hallucination because the person's mind is misinterpreting a real object. In the case of hallucinations, people are sensing or experiencing something that is not really there.

Other prodromal symptoms may be more similar to depression or anxiety than psychosis. For example, prodromal symptoms may include anxiety, declining performance in school or on the job, depressed mood, difficulty sleeping, irritability, and pulling away from significant others. Even though these things may have happened in the past, it is still important to learn about prodromal symptoms. This is because the same prodromal symptoms that happened before psychosis first began are often the same symptoms that occur before another episode of psychosis. These early warning signs are discussed in Chapter 9 on Early Warning Signs and Preventing a Relapse.

Putting It All Together

Psychosis is a mental illness syndrome, which consists of signs that others observe and symptoms that people experience. The nine types of symptoms that occur in psychosis described in this chapter include positive symptoms, negative symptoms, disorganized symptoms, impaired insight, cognitive dysfunction, hostile/aggressive symptoms, catatonic and movement symptoms, mood symptoms and anxiety, and suicidal thoughts. The most obvious symptoms are positive symptoms, or things that have been added to a person's experience, such as delusions or hallucinations. The second major category of symptoms are negative symptoms, or things that have been subtracted from a person's experience, such as social isolation or apathy. These symptoms should not be mistaken for laziness or attitude problems. Even though there are common symptoms, everyone's experience of and types of symptoms will be different.

Symptoms of psychosis can be very scary for those experiencing them and for their families and friends. People experiencing symptoms may not understand their illness or may have impaired insight. They also may despair and give up hope when experiencing an episode. Family and friends should take threats of suicide very seriously as people with psychosis are at a greater risk for attempting and completing suicide than others.

Milder symptoms experienced before the first episode of psychosis are known as prodromal symptoms. These symptoms are important to remember because they usually are the same ones that occur right before another episode. Symptoms, whether in the past or present, are important to discuss with the mental health professional. Family members and friends are very important sources of information for mental health professionals. In the same way, mental health professionals are very important sources of information for patients, family members, and friends. Not only can family and friends provide information to mental health professionals about early symptoms and behaviors, but they also can report how symptoms are changing over time, including when they are improving or getting worse. Mental health professionals can also explain symptoms to families and report on the changes that they are seeing. The following worksheet will help you record and keep track of the symptoms that the patient experienced in the past or currently. It is also a place to keep comments and questions that you wish to discuss with the mental health professional.

Worksheet 2.1 Symptoms Checklist

Symptoms. Place a check next to symptoms experienced.	✓	Observations /Comments. Record when symptoms happened and any questions or comments you may have.
Positive Symptoms		
Hallucinations		
Delusions		
Suspiciousness/Paranoia		
Ideas of Reference		
Bizarre Behavior		
Negative Symptoms		
Anhedonia		
Apathy		
Blunted or Flat Affect		
Emotional Withdrawal		
Low Drive or Motivation		
Poor Grooming/Hygiene		
Slow or Empty Thinking and Speech		

(*continued*)

Worksheet 2.1 Continued

Symptoms. Place a check next to symptoms experienced.	✓	Observations /Comments. Record when symptoms happened and any questions or comments you may have.
Slow Movements		
Social Isolation		
Disorganized Symptoms		
Derailment/Loosening of Associations		
Poverty of Speech Content		
Thought Blocking		
Disorganized Behavior		
Self-Awareness/Insight		
Impaired Insight		
Cognitive Dysfunction		
Difficulties with Abstract Thinking		
Poor Attention and Concentration		
Impaired Information Processing		
Difficulties with Language		
Difficulties with Memory		
Difficulties with Planning		
Aggressiveness		
Increased Hostility or Aggression		

(continued)

33

Worksheet 2.1 Continued

Symptoms. Place a check next to symptoms experienced.	✓	Observations /Comments. Record when symptoms happened and any questions or comments you may have.
Catatonic and Movement Symptoms		
Catatonia		
Abnormal Movements or Posturing		
Mood Symptoms and Suicidal Thoughts		
Depression		
Manic Symptoms		
Anxiety		
Suicidal Thoughts or Behaviors		

Key Chapter Points

☛ Most mental illnesses cause both symptoms that patients experience and signs that doctors or others observe.

☛ Early psychosis is a syndrome that causes many different symptoms.

☛ Nine types of symptoms that may happen during early psychosis include positive symptoms, negative symptoms, disorganized symptoms, impaired insight, cognitive dysfunction, hostile/aggressive symptoms, catatonic and movement symptoms, mood symptoms and anxiety, and suicidal thoughts.

☛ The most outwardly apparent symptoms of psychosis are positive symptoms, which include hallucinations, delusions, suspiciousness/paranoia, and ideas of reference.

☛ Impaired insight, or unawareness of illness, is one of the most difficult problems in psychosis.

☛ The prodromal symptoms that happened before psychosis began are often the same symptoms that occur before another episode of psychosis.

☛ Family and friends should take any expression of suicidal thoughts very seriously because people who have experienced psychosis are at a higher risk for suicide attempts and completed suicide.

Acknowledgments: This chapter was initially developed and written by Tandrea Carter, PhD. Philip D. Harvey, PhD, served as a collaborator for this chapter.

3

What Diagnoses Are Associated with Psychosis?

As described in Chapter 1, psychosis is a syndrome. This syndrome can include a number of different signs and symptoms (see Chapter 2 on What Are the Symptoms of Psychosis?). In this chapter, we discuss the different diagnoses that may relate to psychosis. A diagnosis is a specific medical term given to an illness or syndrome by health-care providers. When a doctor evaluates someone experiencing psychosis, he or she gathers as much information as possible. This information comes from a detailed psychiatric interview and observations, medical records, additional information from family members, a physical exam, cognitive assessments, lab tests, and other types of evaluations to determine the illness underlying the episode of psychosis (see Chapter 5 on The Initial Evaluation of Psychosis).

While gathering information to evaluate a first episode of psychosis, the doctor often comes up with a **differential diagnosis**. This is a list of the most likely reasons for the syndrome, in this case, psychosis. Doctors generally use a differential diagnosis to list the possible illness underlying any health problem. For example, if you go to the doctor for a fever, the doctor may make a list of possible reasons for the fever, such as a minor nose cold caused by a virus, strep throat caused by bacteria, pneumonia, meningitis, or other infections. To narrow down this list to the most likely diagnosis, the doctor then uses information from the history (asking questions), physical exam, and lab tests. Oftentimes a doctor uses a **working diagnosis** to guide treatment planning even if he or she has yet to decide on a final diagnosis.

It is important for patients and families to recognize that making a specific diagnosis often requires long-term information that often is not fully available when a person first comes in for treatment. Being unsure about the diagnosis is one reason why a differential diagnosis and a working diagnosis are so important. A working diagnosis allows the doctor to begin an effective treatment plan even though a final diagnosis may not yet be clear. Some patients and families may want to get a specific diagnosis and may be skeptical when the doctor cannot yet definitively provide one. However, it is important to recognize that one can effectively treat the syndrome of psychosis without having a certain specific diagnosis. This chapter focuses on the three categories that are commonly part of the differential diagnosis of first-episode psychosis.

Three Causes of Psychotic Symptoms

It is important to understand what causes the signs and symptoms of the syndrome of psychosis. If the doctor can determine what causes psychosis, he or she can decide what treatment is best. The three main categories of causes of psychosis are: (1) medical causes, (2) substances, and (3) psychiatric illnesses. We briefly describe each of these types of causes in the following pages.

> If the doctor can determine what causes psychosis, he or she can decide what treatment is best. The three main categories of causes of psychosis are: (1) medical causes, (2) substances, and (3) psychiatric illnesses.

Medical Causes of Psychosis

In rare instances, a physical health condition can cause psychosis. This is a *Psychotic Disorder Due to a General Medical Condition*. In this diagnosis, medical conditions directly cause hallucinations or delusions. Several physical health conditions can cause psychotic symptoms. To find out if such a medical condition is causing the psychosis, a doctor will do several things. First, the doctor will ask questions about the patient's physical health. Then, he or she will do a physical exam. The doctor also may do lab tests and other types of tests.

One example of a physical health problem that may cause psychosis is a brain tumor. To find out if a patient has a brain tumor, the doctor will ask about symptoms that happen when one has a tumor. Then he or she will do a physical exam to check for signs of a brain tumor. If the doctor believes that a tumor may be causing the psychosis, he or she will recommend that the patient get an X-ray of the brain, such as a CAT scan, also called a CT scan. If the scan shows a tumor, then the doctor may conclude that this medical condition is the cause of the psychosis. The doctor would then refer the patient to a neurologist and neurosurgeon to treat the brain tumor.

Table 3.1 lists some of the medical conditions that can sometimes cause psychosis. It is important for doctors to rule out these medical conditions because if the psychosis is in fact coming from one of these disorders, they may need to use very specific medical treatments. For example, doctors use an antibiotic, such as penicillin, to treat neurosyphilis, and an anticonvulsant medicine, which prevents seizures, to treat temporal lobe epilepsy. If there is no evidence that a medical condition is causing the symptoms, then the doctor will decide whether the cause of the psychosis is drug-induced or psychiatric.

Psychosis Caused by Substances

Psychosis caused by a drug or medicine is called a *Substance-Induced Psychotic Disorder*. Many substances can cause psychotic symptoms.

Table 3.1 Some of the Medical Conditions that Can
Sometimes Cause Psychosis

- Addison's disease
- Brain infection
- Brain tumor
- Cushing's disease
- Epilepsy
- Fluid or electrolyte imbalance
- HIV/AIDS
- Huntington's disease
- Hypoxia
- Kidney diseases
- Liver diseases
- Multiple sclerosis
- Neurosyphilis
- Parathyroid diseases (hyperparathyroidism or hypoparathyroidism)
- Parkinson's disease
- Stroke
- Systemic lupus erythematosus
- Temporal lobe epilepsy
- Thyroid disease (hyperthyroidism or hypothyroidism)

Table 3.2 Some of the Drugs of Abuse
that Can Cause Psychosis

- Cocaine
- Ketamine
- Lysergic acid diethylamide (LSD)
- Marijuana
- Methamphetamine
- Phencyclidine (PCP)

To find out if a substance is causing psychosis, the doctor will ask about the patient's contact with certain substances and do lab tests to see if these are in the patient's body. Table 3.2 lists some of the addictive substances (drugs of abuse) that can sometimes cause psychosis.

Other drugs, such as alcohol or addictive sleeping pills, may cause psychosis during withdrawal from the drug. In addition to these addictive drugs of abuse, some medicines can cause psychosis. For example, medical steroids, such as prednisone (Deltasone) and dexamethasone (Decadron), may rarely cause psychosis. Methylphenidate (Ritalin), which is a treatment for attention-deficit/hyperactivity disorder usually in children and adolescents, may cause psychosis at high doses. A number of other medicines, including some of the ones used to treat HIV/AIDS, Parkinson's disease, as well as some other diseases, may cause psychosis in rare instances.

If a lab test shows that one or more of these substances is in the patient's body, then the doctor will recommend that the patient stop using these substances. If a medicine appears to be causing the psychosis, he or she will work with the patient's medical doctor to change the medicine. It may take several days for the substance of abuse or medicine to wash out of the patient's body. If the substance is causing the psychosis, the psychotic symptoms will usually go away when it is gone from the body. If the substance is not causing the psychosis, the psychotic symptoms will continue even when the substances are gone from the body. If the doctor does not believe that a medical condition or a substance is causing the symptoms, then he or she will decide that the cause of the psychosis is most likely psychiatric.

It can sometimes be very challenging to determine whether the psychosis is drug-induced or of a psychiatric origin. Some substances, such as marijuana, may be partly responsible for the onset of a psychotic illness even though the symptoms do not go away when the substance is no longer present (see Chapter 4 on What Causes Primary Psychotic Disorders Like Schizophrenia?). Thus, it is often unclear whether substance use is a trigger for a primary psychotic disorder such as schizophrenia (see next section) or whether the illness is a substance-induced psychotic disorder. Again, the lack of clear diagnosis can sometimes be disappointing or frustrating for patients, their family members, and their doctors alike. However, as noted previously, it is possible to start effective treatment for the syndrome of psychosis without having a certain specific diagnosis. The diagnosis usually becomes clearer as some time passes.

Psychiatric Causes of Psychosis

When there is neither a medical condition nor substance that appears to be causing the psychotic symptoms, the doctor may conclude that the patient's symptoms are psychiatric in origin. This means that the symptoms are coming from a brain disturbance that may be treated by psychiatrists. At this time, there are no lab tests or other medical tests that can prove a psychiatric disorder. So, unlike detecting a medical condition through a medical test or finding a substance in one's body through a urine or blood test, the evaluation of psychiatric disorders depends heavily on a detailed interview and observations. That is, the doctor talks to the patient about recent symptoms and gathers information from the patient and his or her family members about changes in feelings, thoughts, and behaviors. Several types of psychiatric illnesses can lead to the syndrome of psychosis, so the doctor will develop a differential diagnosis, or the most likely reasons for psychosis (see Table 3.3). He or she may need to decide on a working diagnosis before a final diagnosis becomes clear.

Doctors use two sources for classifying psychiatric disorders. One is the **Diagnostic and Statistical Manual of Mental Disorders (DSM)**, which is currently in its fourth edition. The other is the **International Classification of Diseases (ICD)**, which is currently in its tenth edition. Both the DSM and the ICD provide doctors with specific definitions of psychiatric disorders. This allows all doctors to consistently use the same diagnosis when referring to a specific syndrome. As a result, DSM and ICD provide consistent definitions for psychiatric illnesses around the world. So, for example, the definition for schizophrenia is the same in North America, Europe, and Australia. This is especially

Table 3.3 Diagnoses Associated with Psychosis

Psychotic Disorder Due to a General Medical Condition (See Table 3.1)

Substance-Induced Psychotic Disorder (See Table 3.2)

Primary Psychotic Disorders
- Brief psychotic disorder
- Schizophreniform disorder
- Schizophrenia
- Schizoaffective disorder
- Delusional disorder
- Shared psychotic disorder
- Psychotic disorder not otherwise specified

Other Disorders that May Cause Psychosis or Psychotic-Like Symptoms
- Postpartum psychosis
- Major depression
- Bipolar disorder
- Schizotypal personality disorder
- Delirium
- Dementia

important because the exact causes of most psychiatric illnesses are still unclear. So, rather than defining a mental illness by the exact cause, mental health professionals use signs and symptoms to classify the illness. Next, we describe a number of psychiatric disorders, based on detailed definitions found in the DSM.

Primary Psychotic Disorders

One group of psychiatric disorders that cause psychosis is the **primary psychotic disorders**. Doctors call them this because they primarily cause psychosis, rather than depression, anxiety, or another type of syndrome. The most common of these is schizophrenia followed by other disorders closely related to schizophrenia. The seven primary psychotic disorders include brief psychotic disorder, schizophreniform disorder, schizophrenia, schizoaffective disorder, delusional disorder, shared psychotic disorder, and psychotic disorder not otherwise specified.

One group of psychiatric disorders that cause psychosis is the primary psychotic disorders. Doctors call them this because they primarily cause psychosis, rather than depression, anxiety, or another type of syndrome. The most common of these is schizophrenia followed by other disorders closely related to schizophrenia.

1. Brief Psychotic Disorder. People diagnosed with a brief psychotic disorder have one or more positive symptoms (hallucinations or delusions) or disorganized speech or behavior, but these symptoms last only one day to one month. Functioning then returns to normal. Brief psychotic disorder may sometimes happen after a very stressful event, such as the loss of a loved one or being in war or combat. This disorder is uncommon, but when it does happen, it is most likely to happen when a person is between the ages of 20 and 40 years. So, while someone with a brief psychotic disorder has similar symptoms to schizophrenia, the symptoms clear up rapidly and do not return. It is a single psychotic episode that does not recur.

2. Schizophreniform Disorder. People diagnosed with schizophreniform disorder have a combination of psychotic symptoms that last at least one month but do not continue for more than six months. The combination of symptoms may include two or more of the following: delusions, hallucinations, disorganized speech, disorganized or catatonic behavior, and negative symptoms (see Chapter 2 on What Are the Symptoms of Psychosis?). So, schizophreniform disorder is a psychotic episode that lasts longer than brief psychotic disorder, but does not last long enough to receive a diagnosis of schizophrenia.

3. Schizophrenia. People with schizophrenia have a combination of psychotic symptoms as described in Chapter 2. Specifically, schizophrenia is defined by the presence of two or more of the following: delusions, hallucinations, disorganized speech, disorganized or catatonic behavior, and negative symptoms, and the illness lasts for at least six months. So, schizophrenia is very similar to schizophreniform disorder except that in schizophrenia, symptoms last longer. In fact, schizophrenia usually lasts for a very long time and may even be lifelong. People with schizophrenia often need some form of treatment long-term. When a person with schizophrenia continues with his or her treatment (see Chapter 8 on Follow-up and Sticking with Treatment), the symptoms often do not get worse and may get much better. In fact, the positive symptoms often respond quite well to treatment, as described in Chapter 6 on Medicines Used to Treat Psychosis. Some people who continue treatment are able to have good lives with steady jobs and happy relationships, the goal of the **recovery model** (see Chapter 11 on Promoting Recovery). The recovery model aims to empower the patient to achieve his or her own goals for treatment and recovery by actively participating in treatment decisions.

People all over the world have schizophrenia. About 1 in every 100 persons develops schizophrenia during their lifetime. In other words, over the course of one's lifetime the risk of having schizophrenia is about 1%. Schizophrenia affects men and women approximately equally, though recent research suggests that it may be slightly more common in men. The symptoms of schizophrenia usually first become apparent in men between the ages of 20 and 30, and in women between the ages of 24 and 34. However, people who are younger or older also may develop the illness. In fact, "childhood-onset schizophrenia" has been defined by some as development of the illness before the age of 12, and "late-onset schizophrenia" is considered to be the development of the illness after the age of 40.

> People all over the world have schizophrenia. About 1 in every 100 persons develops schizophrenia during their lifetime.

At first, family and friends may think that someone developing psychotic symptoms is "going through a phase." They may not notice the earliest signs and symptoms. But after a while, the symptoms become more obvious. For example, the person may have unusual beliefs, no longer be interested in work or school, have outbursts of anger, stop bathing regularly, or talk to him- or herself.

There are five subtypes of schizophrenia. Each has a different set of symptoms.

- **Schizophrenia—paranoid type** means that the person's symptoms mainly consist of delusions and/or auditory hallucinations. Friends and relatives of the individual may not observe other types of symptoms, like disorganized speech, disorganized behavior, catatonia, flat affect, or inappropriate affect. There also may be minimal cognitive dysfunction in this subtype. Schizophrenia—paranoid type (also called **paranoid schizophrenia**) is probably the most common form of schizophrenia.
- The diagnosis of **schizophrenia—disorganized type** means that the person has disorganized speech, disorganized behavior, and flat or inappropriate affect. People around the individual will notice that he or she is "acting strangely" and his or her speech makes little or no sense. It also may seem like he or she does not have any

emotions (flat affect) or that the emotions do not fit the situation (inappropriate affect).

- In **schizophrenia—catatonic type**, the individual has catatonia. Catatonia is a syndrome that affects movements and speech, such that the person does not move, does not speak, or moves his or her body in an awkward way. Fortunately, the catatonic type of schizophrenia is relatively rare.

- A person is diagnosed with **schizophrenia—undifferentiated type** when the doctor is sure that the individual has schizophrenia, but the symptoms do not fit into one of the earlier three types (paranoid type, disorganized type, or catatonic type).

- The final subtype of schizophrenia is **schizophrenia—residual type**. This means that the person has clearly had a psychotic episode diagnosable as schizophrenia in the past, but currently does not have any positive symptoms (like hallucinations or delusions). However, milder forms of symptoms and prominent negative symptoms are still present.

4. Schizoaffective Disorder. People with schizoaffective disorder have a combination of psychotic symptoms as well as serious mood symptoms. The mood symptoms may be like the symptoms seen in clinical depression, also called major depression, or they may be like the symptoms seen in mania, or bipolar disorder. So, there are two types of schizoaffective disorder.

- In **schizoaffective disorder—depressive type**, the person has the symptoms of schizophrenia described earlier, but also has symptoms of depression. These may include feeling sad or depressed, not being as interested in fun or pleasurable things, a decreased or increased appetite, weight loss or weight gain, having difficulty sleeping, sleeping too much, feeling agitated, feeling slow, fatigue, loss of energy, feeling worthless, feeling guilty for no apparent reason, having difficulty concentrating or making decisions, or having thoughts of death or thoughts of committing suicide.

- In **schizoaffective disorder—bipolar type**, the person has the symptoms of schizophrenia, but also has symptoms of mania. These may include thinking too highly of oneself (an inflated self-esteem, also called grandiosity), not needing to sleep due to having enough energy without sleep, being more talkative than usual, talking very rapidly, having racing thoughts, having poor attention, being agitated, engaging in excessive activities, or going on having spending sprees.

Schizoaffective disorder is less common than schizophrenia. It can start at any age but most often starts in a person's 20s or 30s, like schizophrenia. It is likely to interfere with work, school, and relationships. However, people with schizoaffective disorder can do very well in life if they follow the treatment recommendations of their doctors.

5. Delusional Disorder. Delusional disorder is similar to schizophrenia, except the main symptom is a single delusion. For example, the person may be convinced that a famous person is in love with him or her, that someone is following or out to get him or her, or that a medical condition is present when in fact it is not. Delusional disorder is quite rare, but when it does happen, it tends to be somewhat less severe than schizophrenia because many of the other types of symptoms of schizophrenia (like hallucinations, disorganized thinking, negative symptoms, and cognitive dysfunction) are not present.

6. Shared Psychotic Disorder. This is a very rare diagnosis. A person receives a diagnosis of shared psychotic disorder when he or she develops a delusion while in a close relationship with another person who already has a similar established delusion, as in delusional disorder. So, both people share the same delusion.

7. Psychotic Disorder Not Otherwise Specified (NOS). People diagnosed with psychotic disorder NOS have psychotic symptoms but the doctor does not have enough information to make one of the specific diagnoses described earlier. Doctors often use this as a preliminary diagnosis before deciding on a more conclusive diagnosis. Sometimes a person may receive a new, updated diagnosis when the doctor learns more about a person's symptoms and conducts a more detailed evaluation. A person also may receive the diagnosis of psychotic disorder NOS when the syndrome of psychosis is clearly present, but the psychotic symptoms do not seem to fit the descriptions of any other psychotic disorder described earlier.

Other Psychiatric Disorders that Can Cause Psychosis

Several other disorders can bring about psychotic symptoms (or symptoms that are very similar to psychotic symptoms). These disorders include postpartum psychosis, major depressive disorder, bipolar disorder, schizotypal personality disorder, delirium, and dementia.

> Several other disorders can bring about psychotic symptoms (or symptoms that are very similar to psychotic symptoms). These disorders include postpartum psychosis, major depressive disorder, bipolar disorder, schizotypal personality disorder, delirium, and dementia.

Doctors give a diagnosis of **postpartum psychosis** when a woman has psychotic symptoms anytime within the first three months after giving birth. The symptoms usually begin within the first month after the child's birth and usually come on fairly suddenly. Unlike postpartum depression, which involves depressive stymptoms, postpartum psychosis involves having psychotic symptoms, like hallucinations or delusions. Postpartum psychosis usually gets better with treatment.

Major depression, also called major depressive disorder or clinical depression, is when one has been feeling depressed for at least two weeks. A depressive episode may last weeks, months, or even years. Symptoms may include those listed earlier related to schizoaffective disorder-depressive type. These symptoms of depression are: feeling sad or depressed, not being as interested in fun or pleasurable things, a decreased or increased appetite, weight loss or weight gain, having difficulty sleeping, sleeping too much, feeling agitated, feeling slow, fatigue, loss of energy, feeling worthless, feeling guilty for no apparent reason, having difficulty concentrating or making decisions, or having thoughts of death or thoughts of committing suicide.

Major depression is a common psychiatric disorder, much more common than schizophrenia and other primary psychotic disorders. Whereas schizophrenia affects about 1% of people over the course of their lifetime, an episode of major depression may occur in as many as one in four (25% or one-fourth) of all people during their lifetime. In most cases, major depression does not cause psychosis. However, in some instances, when the depression becomes severe, psychotic symptoms may develop. This is "psychotic depression." The psychosis usually clears up and goes away altogether when the individual receives adequate treatment for depression. Such treatments usually include medicines called **antidepressants**, as well as one or more forms of psychotherapy.

A doctor gives a diagnosis of **bipolar disorder** when someone has had one or more episodes of mania. Episodes of major depression may happen in between the episodes of mania. As listed earlier in the description of schizoaffective disorder—bipolar type, symptoms of mania may include thinking too highly of oneself (an inflated self-esteem, also called grandiosity), not needing to sleep due to having enough energy without sleep, being more talkative than usual, talking very rapidly, having racing thoughts, having poor attention, being agitated, engaging in excessive activities, or going on spending sprees. Like major depression, many cases of mania do not cause psychotic symptoms. However, when the manic episode is severe, psychotic symptoms like hallucinations or delusions may develop. Also like psychotic depression, once the mania is adequately treated, the psychosis usually clears up and goes away. Treatments for bipolar disorder include medicine, some of which are **mood stabilizers**, as well as certain types of psychotherapy. Distinguishing between bipolar disorder and schizoaffective disorder—bipolar type is often difficult even for experienced doctors. Often, a working diagnosis is made, and then once more long-term observation and monitoring becomes available, it becomes clearer whether the patient's symptoms are more consistent with bipolar disorder or schizoaffective disorder.

Most doctors think of **schizotypal personality disorder** as a mild form of schizophrenia that never leads to the full syndrome of psychosis. A person with this diagnosis may have strange beliefs or odd behaviors, or be socially withdrawn or uncomfortable with close relationships. The person has had such symptoms or behaviors since he or she was young, and they seem to just be part of the individual's personality. The person may seem odd and eccentric, but the symptoms are not truly psychotic.

Both **delirium** and **dementia** are disorders that cause confusion. That is, people with either of these conditions may not know the date, where they are, or even their name. As a result, the confusion causes **disorientation** (not knowing the time, place, or situation). People with primary psychotic disorders like schizophrenia, or any of the other disorders described earlier, do not have this form of confusion or disorientation. They know who they are, where they are, and what the date is.

Delirium is a state of confusion that develops rapidly, over the course of hours or days. It is usually due to a medical condition, like having had a seizure, having a high fever, or having an infection somewhere in the body. Delirium may also be caused by taking a drug of abuse or even withdrawing from some drugs, like alcohol. It is a medical emergency requiring immediate medical attention to treat the underlying cause of the delirium. Delirium can happen in people of any age. In addition to causing confusion, delirium can sometimes cause psychotic symptoms, like hallucinations.

Dementia also causes confusion and disorientation, but dementia usually develops slowly, over the course of months or years. Dementia usually occurs in older people or the elderly, usually after the age of 65 years, and often after the age of 80. The most common cause of dementia is Alzheimer's disease, though other diseases, such as repeated strokes, Parkinson's disease, or Huntington's disease, may cause dementia as well. In addition to causing confusion, dementia can sometimes cause psychotic symptoms, like hallucinations or delusions.

Putting It All Together

There are several different diagnoses associated with psychosis. The three major categories of causes of psychosis include medical causes, substances, and a number of psychiatric illnesses. Chapter 4 discusses in detail what research has uncovered about the causes of psychiatric illnesses like schizophrenia.

Schizophrenia is one of several primary psychotic disorders, a group of psychiatric disorders that primarily cause psychosis. Other disorders can cause psychotic symptoms or symptoms similar to these but are not considered psychotic disorders. A few examples of such disorders include major depressive disorder, bipolar disorder, and dementia. It is often difficult to make a specific diagnosis when long-term information is not available at first. In instances in which a definitive diagnosis is uncertain, a working diagnosis allows the doctor to begin effective treatments for the psychosis even before a final diagnosis is made.

Key Chapter Points

- ☞ A diagnosis is a specific medical term given to an illness or syndrome by health-care providers.
- ☞ The three main categories of causes of psychosis are: (1) medical causes, (2) substances, and (3) psychiatric illnesses.
- ☞ Sometimes a specific diagnosis is difficult to make initially, so doctors often use a working diagnosis in order to start a treatment plan. It is possible to start effective treatment for the syndrome of psychosis without having a certain specific diagnosis. In these cases, the diagnosis usually becomes clearer as some time passes.
- ☞ To make a diagnosis doctors use information from detailed psychiatric interview and observations, other records and collateral information, a physical exam, cognitive assessments, lab tests, and other types of evaluations to determine the cause of an episode of psychosis.
- ☞ When deciding on the final diagnosis, doctors use two classifications, the DSM and ICD, which give detailed, standard definitions for each psychiatric disorder.
- ☞ The seven primary psychotic disorders include brief psychotic disorder, schizophreniform disorder, schizophrenia, schizoaffective disorder, delusional disorder, shared psychotic disorder, and psychotic disorder not otherwise specified.
- ☞ Other psychiatric disorders that can bring about psychotic symptoms (or symptoms that are very similar to psychotic symptoms) include postpartum psychosis, major depressive disorder, bipolar disorder, schizotypal personality disorder, delirium, and dementia.

Acknowledgments: This chapter was initially developed by Amy S. Leiner, PhD. Ross M.G. Norman, PhD, served as a collaborator for this chapter.

4 What Causes Primary Psychotic Disorders Like Schizophrenia?

Doctors and researchers have been able to identify the causes of a variety of medical conditions, such as the common cold, a heart attack, and gout, to name a few. For example, there are different types of viruses that cause the symptoms of a common cold. By knowing what causes a medical problem, doctors are able to treat the condition in the most focused way possible. In the previous chapter, three general categories of causes of psychosis were presented: (1) medical causes, (2) substances, including certain drugs of abuse and several medicines, and (3) a number of psychiatric illnesses. This chapter presents what is currently known about the causes of the third of these, psychiatric illnesses, especially primary psychotic disorders like schizophrenia.

Some health conditions have a single, straight-forward cause. As mentioned earlier, a common cold is caused by a virus. However, many illnesses do not have a single identifiable cause. Rather, they are caused by a combination of **risk factors**. A risk factor is any event, exposure, or entity that occurs before the illness and that research has shown plays a role in causing the illness. For example, cigarette smoking is a well-known risk factor for lung cancer. Smoking occurs before the lung cancer develops, and researchers have proven that smoking cigarettes plays a part in causing many cases of lung cancer. Because schizophrenia and related psychotic disorders are such complex illnesses, it is sometimes unclear if some of the risk factors truly occur before the illness. Some risk factors may make some people more psychosis-prone (see Chapter 1). In other words, some risk factors are best thought of as increasing one's tendency towards psychosis rather than actually causing psychosis.

Over the past several decades, researchers have identified some of the likely causes of complex medical conditions like diabetes, high blood pressure, and psychosis. For each of these, as is true of most medical conditions, there is no single cause. Rather, a number of risk factors, both internal (like certain genes) and external (like exposures that stress the body, such as stressful life events or drugs) combine in complex ways to bring about the illness. Research is showing that some genes may only increase one's risk for schizophrenia when certain external exposures are also present. For example, some research studies suggest that one particular gene that may increase risk for schizophrenia only seems to do so in people who smoked marijuana during adolescence.

Psychotic disorders are not the result of a single cause like the virus that causes the symptoms of a common cold. Instead, a combination of risk factors cause psychosis. This chapter first briefly describes the important role of genes as a cause of primary psychotic disorders like schizophrenia and then a number of risk factors occurring early in life (during pregnancy/delivery and in infancy). The combination of certain genes and a number of these early-life risk factors probably leads to abnormal early brain development, which sets the stage for the later development of psychosis. Then we describe other risk factors that may occur during childhood and adolescence, which bring about further abnormal brain development during adolescence. This combination of genes, early-life risk factors, later risk factors, and abnormal brain development ultimately may lead to the onset of psychosis. As explained at the end of the chapter, this way of viewing the cause of schizophrenia and related disorders is consistent with the two models discussed in Chapter 1, the neurodevelopmental model and the diathesis-stress model.

> Psychotic disorders are not the result of a single cause
> like the virus that causes the symptoms of a common cold.
> Instead, a combination of risk factors cause psychosis.

Genes

Most people with a primary psychotic disorder like schizophrenia do not have any relatives with the illness. However, research has shown that the more closely related someone is to a person with a psychotic disorder, the more likely they are to develop a similar illness. First-degree relatives of someone with psychosis (parents, siblings, and children) have a higher risk of developing psychosis than people who are not relatives of someone with psychosis. As mentioned in the previous chapter, the lifetime risk of developing schizophrenia is about 1%. That is, 1 in 100 people will develop schizophrenia over the course of a lifetime. For people with a first-degree relative with schizophrenia, like a mother, father, sister, or brother, this risk goes up to approximately 15%. Research also has shown that among twins, if one twin has schizophrenia, an identical twin is much more likely to also develop schizophrenia (about 50% or one-half chance) compared to a fraternal twin (about 15% chance). This information indicates that psychosis is **heritable**, which means that it is partly caused by genes. **Genes** are segments of DNA that pass along the "blueprints" of how the body's cells are to make proteins. Proteins, in turn, form the building blocks for all parts of the body, including the brain.

Researchers now know that a large portion of the cause of schizophrenia, approximately 80–85%, comes from genes (see Figure 4.1). It is unlikely that only one gene can cause psychosis. Rather, a number of genes probably each play a small role in a person's likelihood of developing psychosis. It may be the combination of a number of these **risk genes** that accounts for the genetic portion of the cause of schizophrenia. Researchers are working to determine the exact genes that increase risk for schizophrenia. To date, they have found a number of **candidate genes** (genes that have a strong possibility of being risk genes). For example, some of these candidate genes are genes that affect the dopamine and glutamate systems in the brain, which are described later. However, more research is required to prove which genes play a role in causing schizophrenia and which do not. Also, because genes serve as the "blueprints" for cells to make specific proteins, more research is needed to better understand the role of specific proteins in the development of the disorder.

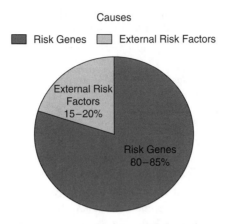

Figure 4.1 The Causes of Primary Psychotic Disorders Such as Schizophrenia

> Researchers now know that a large portion of the cause of schizophrenia, approximately 80–85%, comes from genes. It is unlikely that only one gene can cause psychosis. Rather, a number of genes probably each play a small role in a person's likelihood of developing psychosis.

Risk Factors that Occur before Birth, during Delivery, and in Infancy

As mentioned earlier, a number of risk factors may combine to bring about psychosis. Many of these risk factors are the risk genes that make up a large portion of the cause of psychosis. However, some risk factors are nongenetic, meaning that they are not due to one's genes. It is estimated that 15–20% (or about one-fifth) of the cause of schizophrenia is driven by these external risk factors. Some of these risk factors occur very early in life, before birth, during delivery, or in infancy. A few of these are shown in Table 4.1.

Abnormalities in Early Brain Development

Researchers believe that the combination of risk genes and external risk factors that may occur early in life leads to abnormalities in early

Table 4.1 Early-life Risk Factors (Risk Factors that
Occur before Birth, during Delivery, and in Infancy)

- Nutritional deficiency in the mother during pregnancy
- Exposure of the mother to a severe stressor during pregnancy
- Infections in the mother during pregnancy (such as influenza)
- Rh blood-type incompatibility between the mother and fetus
- Pregnancy and delivery complications
- Low birth weight
- Brain infections during infancy

brain development (see Figure 4.2). These abnormalities in brain development may even occur before birth, during fetal brain development.

Genes are important in the development of the brain. They control the growth and development of cells in the brain. These cells are called **neurons**. Genes provide neurons with a "blueprint" of how to make proteins that support the structure and function of the brain. Certain genes make **neurotransmitters**, or the substances needed for communication between neurons. Also, there are specific genes that tell neurons when to grow and how to change.

Doctors now know that illnesses like psychosis have their roots in brain dysfunction. Researchers have found abnormalities in brain structure and function in people with psychosis. The size of particular areas of the brain, like the lateral ventricles and hippocampus, is slightly different in individuals with psychosis compared to those without psychosis. Studies have shown that people with psychosis have abnormal patterns of activity in particular brain regions, including the frontal cortex. There also appear to be abnormalities in the neurotransmitters that allow neurons to communicate. This leads to altered communication among cells in the brain. For example, individuals with psychosis seem to have higher levels of the neurotransmitter **dopamine** in some parts of the brain and lower levels in other parts. Individuals with psychosis also have altered brain levels of other neurotransmitters, such as **glutamate**.

The abnormalities in brain development that occur early in life among people who later develop psychosis are very subtle. They usually remain undetected. The above changes in neurons and neurotransmitters have only been discovered through research with people who have already developed a psychotic illness like schizophrenia.

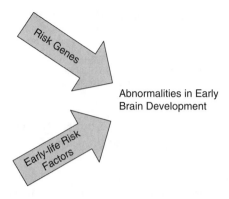

Abnormalities in Early
Brain Development

Figure 4.2 Abnormalities in Early Brain Development

Risk Factors Occurring during Childhood and Adolescence

The abnormalities in early brain development usually do not lead to psychosis during childhood or early adolescence. Rather, psychosis usually first begins in late adolescence or young adulthood. However, research has shown that most children who later develop schizophrenia do have some difficulties early in life. For example, they may have poor motor coordination, minor decreases in intelligence or IQ (intelligence quotient) compared to what would be expected, and subtle difficulties in social adjustment. These difficulties may lead to declining grades in school. Children who later develop schizophrenia are also more likely to have depression and social anxiety than children who do not develop schizophrenia. People who later develop psychosis also may have experienced minor psychotic-like experiences during childhood and adolescence. These are like the schizotypal or psychotic-like symptoms described in the continuum of psychosis presented in Chapter 1.

Some risk factors for psychosis may occur during childhood and adolescence. These risk factors may not lead to any problems in most people. However, for those who already have early brain abnormalities because of a combination of risk genes and early-life risk factors, these additional risk factors during childhood and adolescence may ultimately bring about schizophrenia. Some of these risk factors are shown in Table 4.2. For example, various **stressful life events** may be

Table 4.2 Risk Factors Happening during
Childhood and Adolescence

- Child abuse
- Ethnic segregation and discrimination
- Social adversity (such as poverty)
- Marijuana use during adolescence

a risk factor for schizophrenia. Such difficulties may include child abuse, discrimination, poverty, and the sense of "social defeat" that these problems may lead to.

Another external factor that may be a risk factor for schizophrenia and other primary psychotic disorders is substance abuse during adolescence. Research suggests that adolescent drug use, especially marijuana use, increases one's risk of developing psychosis. The main active ingredients in marijuana may affect the brain systems (for example, the dopamine neurotransmitter system) that are affected in schizophrenia. Most adolescents who use marijuana do not develop schizophrenia. However, for those with a combination of risk genes and early-life risk factors, using marijuana may be a dangerous "second hit" to an already at-risk brain.

> Research suggests that adolescent drug use, especially marijuana use, increases one's risk of developing psychosis.

Abnormalities in Brain Development during Adolescence

Individuals who develop a psychotic disorder usually experience their first episode of psychosis between the ages of 16 and 30 years. However, some may show signs as early as middle school, while other people will not display psychotic symptoms until their 30s.

Adolescence is an important period in the development of the brain. As the adolescent brain develops, young people experience development in social, psychological, and educational areas. Coping skills mature. Many adolescents describe this period as being particularly stressful because of all of the changes that come along with the move towards independence and adulthood. Adolescents also experience many social pressures during this time, such as doing well in school and making friends. For someone whose genes and early-life risk factors put them at risk for psychosis, these pressures may interact with normal hormonal changes of adolescence to bring about subtle brain abnormalities and problems in the dopamine system.

Individuals who develop psychosis often display slight signs during adolescence. These signs may include mood changes, anxiety, irritability, mild positive symptoms (such as magical thinking, suspiciousness, and odd beliefs), social withdrawal, and cognitive dysfunction. These slight signs, which comprise the prodromal phase, often last several years before the onset of psychosis (see Chapter 9 on Early Warning Signs and Preventing a Relapse). People who later develop psychosis also often experience mild learning problems or school difficulties in childhood and adolescence. These are mild forms of the cognitive dysfunction (such as problems with attention, learning, memory, and planning) described in Chapter 2 (What Are the Symptoms of Psychosis?).

Research suggests that in addition to the abnormalities that occur in early brain development (for example, during fetal growth and infancy), abnormalities may also occur during the important period of adolescent brain maturation (see Figure 4.3). In addition to the abnormalities in neurons and neurotransmitters described earlier, other abnormalities may occur. There may be abnormalities in the connections between neurons. That is, a normal process of **pruning** occurs in

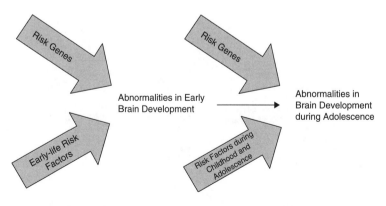

Figure 4.3 Abnormalities in Brain Development during Adolescence

childhood and adolescence to optimize these connections. Synaptic pruning produces more efficient connections in the brain by reducing the number of "weak" connections between neurons. Abnormalities of the pruning process during adolescent development may be under genetic control, but risk factors that happen during adolescence may also affect it.

Putting It All Together

So far, we have described a series of events, which usually occurs quietly without recognition or any idea that a primary psychotic disorder may be developing. School difficulties and social problems may develop during childhood and adolescence, so the developing illness is not completely silent during this early stage. But these common problems do not usually prompt parents to seek psychiatric evaluation until more obvious symptoms have appeared.

This series of events includes a combination of risk genes, early-life risk factors, abnormalities in early brain development, risk factors during childhood and adolescence, and abnormalities in brain development during adolescence. Researchers currently believe that this is the likely path towards the brain dysfunction that leads to the signs and symptoms of psychosis.

This series of events is consistent with two models that were mentioned in Chapter 1, the neurodevelopmental model and the diathesis-stress model. That is, as shown in Figure 4.4, psychosis comes about

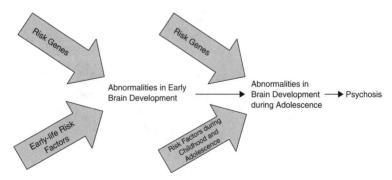

Figure 4.4 The Likely Path toward Developing Psychosis

due to a cascade of events occurring during neurodevelopment, or brain development. Also as shown in Figure 4.4, the cause of psychosis is related to both genetic risk ("diathesis"), as well as external risk factors during childhood and adolescence ("stress").

Key Chapter Points

- ☛ By knowing what causes medical problems, doctors are able to treat them in the best way possible.
- ☛ Doctors now know that illnesses like psychosis have their roots in brain dysfunction.
- ☛ The combination of certain genes and a number of early-life risk factors probably leads to abnormal early brain development, which sets the stage for the later development of psychosis.
- ☛ It is unlikely that only one gene can cause psychosis. Instead, a number of genes each play a small role in a person's risk for developing psychosis.
- ☛ The abnormal brain development that happens early in life among people who later develop psychosis is very slight and usually remains undetected and quiet.
- ☛ In addition to the abnormal early brain development, abnormalities may also happen during the important period of adolescent brain maturation.
- ☛ Research suggests that adolescent drug use, especially marijuana use, increases one's risk of developing psychosis.

Acknowledgments: This chapter was initially developed by Kevin D. Tessner, PhD. Matthew R. Broome, MRCPsych, PhD, served as a collaborator for this chapter.

II Clarifying the Initial Evaluation and Treatment of Psychosis

5 The Initial Evaluation of Psychosis

People experiencing a first episode of psychosis and their families sometimes hesitate in seeking mental health evaluation and treatment. One reason may be that they do not know what to expect. In addition, old wives' tales, stories from the media, or other ideas about what happens to people with psychosis may be frightening. This chapter explains the **evaluation** provided in a health-care setting when people seek help for a first psychotic episode.

A thorough evaluation is the first step for mental health professionals to help people experiencing a first psychotic episode. The main reason for evaluation is to better understand what people with psychosis are experiencing. Just like medical illnesses, early psychosis differs greatly across individuals. It can include many different types of signs and symptoms (see Chapter 2) that are caused by a number of different disorders (see Chapter 3). So, a thorough evaluation allows the mental health professional to compile all sorts of information, from different perspectives, to arrive at the most appropriate diagnosis and develop the most effective treatment plan.

As described in Chapter 3, a thorough evaluation assesses three types of possible causes of psychosis. Are the psychotic symptoms a result of a medical condition that requires treatment? Are they stemming from a substance of abuse? Or, do they indicate a psychiatric illness, such as major depression, bipolar disorder, or a primary psychotic disorder? Importantly, the evaluation can provide families with an explanation

> A thorough evaluation is the first step for mental health professionals to help people experiencing their first psychotic episode. The main reason for evaluation is to better understand what people with psychosis are experiencing. Just like medical illnesses, early psychosis differs greatly across individuals.

for what their loved one is experiencing. It also may help the person with psychosis to feel better understood (see Figure 5.1).

This chapter describes the typical evaluation that is provided when someone first comes into a mental health facility with psychosis. Most importantly, interviews and observations allow the mental health professional to understand the nature of the psychotic symptoms, including when they started, how they progressed, etc. In addition to gathering information from the patient, the mental health professional will want to collect any other records that may be helpful and to contact others who know the patient to get their perspectives. The mental health professional will usually do a number of medical and

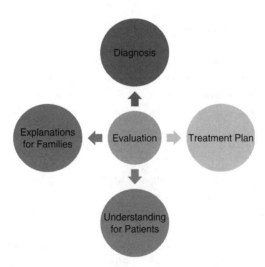

Figure 5.1 Evaluation Provides a Diagnosis, Explanations for Families, and Understanding for Patients, and Helps to Form a Treatment Plan

psychological exams, including a physical exam, cognitive assessments, lab tests, and perhaps an electroencephalogram and an imaging study. Each of these tests is described in the following pages.

Before we explain the parts of the evaluation process, it is important to understand the difference between **inpatient** and **outpatient** evaluation and treatment settings. Inpatient settings are usually in hospitals, and patients usually stay overnight for several days. The amount of time spent depends on how serious the individual's symptoms are. Patients in an outpatient setting visit the treatment facility for an appointment, but then return home. Whether the evaluation needs to be done in an inpatient or outpatient setting is usually determined by the mental health professional, the family, and the patient, based on many factors, including how serious the psychotic symptoms are. We return to the inpatient versus outpatient settings at the end of this chapter.

Interviews and Observations

The initial interview (discussion between the patient and the mental health professional) and behavioral observations (watching the patient's movements and behaviors during the interview) are often done by a **psychiatrist** or a **psychologist**. A psychiatrist is a doctor who has received training in medicine. Psychiatrists evaluate and treat people with mental illnesses and often prescribe medicines as part of the treatment. A psychologist is similar to a psychiatrist, but has received training in the field of psychology rather than in medicine. Although psychologists are usually not licensed to prescribe medicines, they have other skills, such as performing formal psychological testing (like the cognitive assessments described later in this chapter). However, not all mental health professionals are doctors. Other mental health professionals include psychiatric nurses, social workers, counselors, mental health associates, peer specialists, and other trained staff who work as part of the treatment team with a psychiatrist and a psychologist.

The evaluation process consists of several steps. First, a psychiatrist or psychologist will conduct an **interview** with the patient. This interview helps the mental health professional to understand the difficulties the patient has been experiencing. The doctor will ask many questions to understand these experiences. It is also common for doctors to ask several questions about the patient's family.

The doctor will have a number of questions for people who know the patient well, like his or her family members. All of these questions help address specific symptoms that comprise various diagnoses described in Chapter 3. This large amount of information about what has been going on in the past and more recently is sometimes called the **history**. The mental health professional wants to know what symptoms the patient has experienced and the events that led up to these difficulties. Gathering all of this history includes asking patients questions about any mental illnesses in family members, previous medical conditions or head injuries, recent social functioning, past academic performance, and past and current substance use.

Mental health professionals sometimes use interview guides to organize their questions when taking the history to better understand the symptoms that the patient is experiencing. When conducting the interview, the mental health professional will often take notes to assist in later putting all of the pieces of information together. These notes and the results of all of the testing described in the following pages become part of the patient's **medical record**. The medical record documents the evaluation and treatments that are prescribed. It also helps mental health professionals communicate with one another about the patient's progress. The medical record is confidential, meaning that only health professionals treating the patient have access to it. The laws defining exactly which health professionals and health agencies have access to it vary across states/provinces and countries.

In addition to completing a thorough interview, the mental health professional will observe the patient's behavior. Such **observations** include watching the patient's facial expression, movements, and body language. People that know the patient well, like his or her family members, also may give information about such behaviors. Again, family members are very important sources of information during the initial evaluation.

The doctor doing the interview will also do a **mental status exam** as part of the interview. The mental status exam includes an assessment of several aspects of mental functioning, including: appearance, attitude, behavior, speech, mood, affect, thought process, thought content, insight, judgment, impulse control, and cognition. Each of these is described below and shown in Figure 5.2.

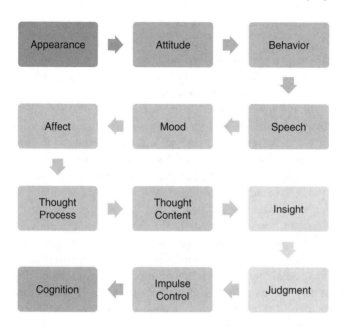

Figure 5.2 Parts of a Mental Status Exam

1. ***Appearance:*** Mental health professionals observe the patient's posture, level of eye contact, and hygiene and grooming. They also look for unusual clothing or hairstyles not typical of the patient's cultural background. Sometimes psychotic symptoms like disorganized thinking and disorganized behavior may lead to an odd appearance. Negative symptoms may make it hard for the patient to maintain appropriate hygiene.

2. ***Attitude:*** They also assess the patient's attitude, or the way he or she engages and participates in the interview. Restlessness, anxiety, tension, suspiciousness, and poor cooperation may reveal clues about specific symptoms.

3. ***Behavior:*** Mental health professionals look for any odd or unusual behaviors. They also will note any unusual movements, including slowness, tics, tremors, or fidgeting. Negative symptoms may cause a slowing of movements. Some psychotic symptoms may lead to unusual movements, postures, or mannerisms.

4. ***Speech:*** Mental health professionals also observe the patient's speech. For example, is the patient's speech abnormally slow or fast? Too loud or soft? Does his or her speech change depending on what he

or she is discussing? Or does it lack these normal changes? Does the patient give an appropriate response to questions?

5. **Mood:** Mental health professionals also assess the patient's mood. For example, is the patient happy or sad? They look for mood symptoms such as depression or mania.

6. **Affect:** Whereas "mood" is one's own report of one's inner emotional state, "affect" refers to the observed emotional state. Affect is assessed by looking at facial expressions, tone of voice, and gestures. In some cases, the individual will report a mood state that does not match with his or her affect. In other cases, the patient's affect may appear to be blunted or flat, as described in the discussion of negative symptoms in Chapter 2.

7. **Thought process:** Mental health professionals ask about and observe the patient's thought process, which is how the thoughts are put together. Psychosis sometimes causes disorganization in the thought process, such as derailment or loosening of associations. A patient may be unaware of disorganized thoughts. However, any disorganization of thinking is often obvious to treatment providers and others who have spent time with the patient.

8. **Thought content:** Unlike the thought process, which refers to *how* the patient thinks, thought content refers to *what* the patient is thinking about. The mental health professional will assess for delusional thoughts, paranoia or suspiciousness, hallucinations, and ideas of reference. Importantly, mental health professionals also almost always ask about suicidal thoughts and thoughts of harming others. These are standard questions asked of most people receiving a mental health evaluation.

9. **Insight:** Insight refers to how well the patient understands his or her illness. Assessing the level of insight may be helpful in estimating how well the individual will engage in treatment and stick with or adhere to the treatment plan (see Chapter 8).

10. **Judgment:** Similar to insight, mental health professionals also examine the patient's judgment. This can give clues about the patient's decision-making ability. Assessing a person's judgment also helps estimate the likelihood of future risky behavior.

11. **Impulse control:** Mental health professionals assess impulse control, or how well a patient is able to stop himself or herself

from participating in dangerous behaviors or acting on impulses. Impulse control also explains how well a patient thinks through decisions.

12. *Cognition:* The mental status exam also includes a review of the patient's cognitive abilities, including attention, memory, planning skills, and reasoning ability.

The many different questions during the interview and mental status exam are important in order to establish a diagnosis and develop a treatment plan. After the interview, behavioral observations, and mental status exam, doctors may carry out other steps in the evaluation process, described in the following pages. The goal of collecting all of this information is to make treatment recommendations that aim for symptom reduction, improvement in the patient's quality of life, and ultimately recovery.

> The goal of collecting all of this information is to make treatment recommendations that aim for symptom reduction, improvement in the patient's quality of life, and ultimately recovery.

Other Records and Collateral Information

Sometimes the evaluation may include gathering information from sources other than the patient. For example, if the patient had academic problems, the mental health professional may ask for school records. Similarly, mental health professionals may want medical records from past doctors. This is especially important if the patient has had earlier mental health evaluation or treatment.

In many cases, patients cannot fully explain their recent history because of symptoms such as impaired insight, paranoia, disorganized thoughts, or poverty of speech. Mental health professionals will try to get **collateral information** from others, such as family members or friends. Collateral information is additional information that may confirm the patient's history or provide another perspective on recent problems. Mental health professionals want this information to get several views on what has been going on.

Physical Exam

Individuals with mental illnesses may have physical illnesses as well. A doctor often completes a physical exam to check for problems that may have led to psychosis. A number of medical illnesses can cause psychosis. Patients in an inpatient setting often receive a physical exam when admitted to the hospital. The physical exam usually includes testing of eye movements, balance, strength in various muscle groups, and reflexes. The doctor will also listen to the patient's heart and lungs with a stethoscope and may look into the patient's eyes and ears with other instruments. Other parts of the physical exam may rule-out the presence of a disease in other parts of the body. In general, the physical exam does not hurt and takes about half an hour.

Cognitive Assessments

Detailed assessments of cognitive functioning are commonly done, especially in research settings. These assessments can be similar to some of the mental status exam questions described earlier, but even more extensive. Some cognitive functions, like attention, learning, memory, and planning, may be assessed with special verbal or written tests. These assessments are important because one's level of cognitive functioning may influence recovery. Cognitive assessment also may identify areas of strengths and weaknesses that are important to consider during treatment planning. Mental health professionals also use these assessments to diagnose some mental disorders or to determine if a patient meets disability requirements.

Lab Tests

When admitted to the hospital for an episode of psychosis, or even in the outpatient setting, doctors first try to rule out any medical or drug-induced causes of psychosis. Drug-induced psychosis might result from drugs like amphetamines, cocaine, LSD, marijuana, or PCP. Doctors use blood and urine tests to check for the presence of drugs and other substances that may cause drug-induced psychosis. Blood tests also check for infections, vitamin deficiencies, thyroid problems, liver diseases, kidney diseases, and neurosyphilis. In some instances, doctors may need to perform a **lumbar puncture** (also called a **spinal tap**) to rule-out an infection in the brain by examining cerebrospinal fluid.

Electroencephalogram

Mental health professionals often ask a neurologist to conduct an **electroencephalogram (EEG)** as part of the first evaluation for psychosis. An EEG records the electrical activity in the brain. To do the EEG, the clinician will attach a number of small electrodes and wires to the person's scalp. The EEG is painless and is commonly used to assess for seizures. Mental health professionals mainly conduct an EEG to rule out rare seizure disorders, like temporal lobe epilepsy, that sometimes cause psychotic-like symptoms. Temporal lobe epilepsy is a type of seizure disorder that can mimic mental illnesses that cause psychosis because it sometimes causes hallucinations or delusions.

Imaging Studies

Although a first episode of psychosis is often due to a psychiatric illness such as a primary psychotic disorder, **imaging studies** (also called **neuroimaging**) are often done. Such studies are used to rule-out other causes of psychosis, like a brain tumor. Imaging studies allow radiologists and mental health professionals to look at the brain to determine if there are any abnormal findings, such as brain tumors or infections.

There are several types of imaging studies. One type is a **computerized axial tomography (CAT) scan**, also called a computerized tomography (CT) scan, which is similar to a very detailed X-ray of the brain. The X-ray is processed by a computer to produce a picture of the inside of the brain. A CT scan mainly looks for brain tumors or other lesions that could cause the psychotic symptoms. A CT scan (rather than one of the other imaging studies described next) is commonly used as part of the initial, or first evaluation because it is relatively inexpensive. Like the other imaging studies, it is painless, and it is also **noninvasive**, meaning it does not involve any needles, incisions, or entry into the body.

Another type of imaging study is the **magnetic resonance imaging (MRI)**. The MRI is another noninvasive procedure that shows doctors the brain structure. This allows them to see any abnormalities, such as tumors, swelling inside the brain, or small areas of disease that might cause psychotic symptoms. The MRI uses magnetic waves instead of X-ray radiation. To have a CT scan or MRI, the patient must lie down

> When admitted to the hospital for an episode of psychosis, or even in the outpatient setting, doctors first try to rule out any medical or drug-induced causes of psychosis.

on a bed-like table, which slides into a large tube. When inside an MRI machine, the patient will hear loud noises from the machine. While it is just the machine at work, these sounds do bother some people. Others also might become claustrophobic or fearful of the enclosed space. But these tests do not take long, and they are often important.

If the initial evaluation and treatment are carried out in a clinical research center, researchers may perform other studies as part of an extensive evaluation. This may include specialized imaging studies. A more specialized type of MRI is the **functional magnetic resonance imaging (fMRI).** Other types of research scans include the **positron emission tomography (PET) scan** and the **single photon emission computed tomography (SPECT) scan.** These special imaging studies that are used for research measure blood flow in the brain, helping to determine how the brain is functioning. Many times, doctors or researchers will ask patients to perform **cognitive tasks** during the fMRI or PET scan. Cognitive tasks include things such as remembering items or putting items into categories. Doctors can determine how different parts of the brain are functioning based on blood flow to those areas.

Combining the Pieces of an Evaluation

The mental health professional uses all of the information gathered from the interview, behavioral observations, mental status exam, other records, collateral information, physical exam, cognitive assessments, lab tests, EEG, and imaging studies to make a diagnosis. As discussed in Chapter 3, this sometimes requires an initial working diagnosis and a differential diagnosis until a more firm diagnosis becomes clear. Once all of the information is gathered and the diagnosis is made, the mental health professional will work with the patient and his or her family to develop a treatment plan. This treatment plan usually involves a medicine, as discussed in Chapter 6, as well as one or more psychosocial interventions, described in Chapter 7.

Sometimes, mental health professionals are limited in what they can discuss with family members if the patient has not provided consent for the mental health professional to do so. It is therefore important for patients to sign all necessary forms to allow for open communication between the mental health professional and close family members. Confidentiality rules and laws may not allow mental health professionals to share patient-specific information if consent is not given. This generally does not apply to life-threatening situations (e.g., suicidal thoughts or actions, serious dangerousness, inability to care for self, or during an emergency evaluation) or for general information-sharing that is not patient-specific (e.g., education about psychosis in general).

Inpatient versus Outpatient Evaluation

As mentioned at the beginning of this chapter, doctors conduct evaluations either in an inpatient or outpatient setting. The level of symptoms and the mental health professional's opinion about the level of care that is needed largely determine where evaluation and treatment should begin. Doctors will recommend hospitalization if the patient poses any possible danger to self or others. They also will recommend hospitalization if the psychosis is serious enough to significantly disrupt the patient's functioning or ability to care for himself or herself.

Inpatient care (in the hospital) can be either voluntary or involuntary. In the case of **voluntary inpatient treatment**, the patient chooses willingly to sign in to the hospital. On the other hand, in **involuntary inpatient treatment**, the patient has symptoms that require hospitalization, but he or she does not agree to sign in to the hospital. A psychiatrist or psychologist can then keep the patient in the hospital, depending on local, state/provincial, or national laws. This is also called **involuntary hospitalization**, **civil commitment**, or **compulsory treatment**. Patients with severe symptoms can be committed from several days to a couple of weeks in most hospital settings. However, commitment can be longer if needed, again depending on local, state/ provincial, or national laws. Once acute psychosis lessens, patients often can switch from an inpatient to an outpatient treatment setting.

In some areas, **outpatient commitment** (also called involuntary community treatment) may be required when the patient would be best served by outpatient treatment, and a court order is issued to ensure that the patient stays in outpatient treatment. If he or she fails to continue outpatient treatment, then hospitalization may be necessary.

Whether in an inpatient or outpatient setting, mental health professionals encourage patients to be in treatment voluntarily. Voluntary treatment strengthens the working relationship between the patient and his or her mental health professionals, and patients have better outcomes when voluntarily engaged in treatment.

Putting It All Together

The evaluation process for psychosis can be frightening for patients and family members. There may be many unknowns and few explanations from busy treatment professionals about this process. In addition, patients with early psychosis are often young (in late adolescence or early adulthood) and may have limited or no experience with hospitals or mental health treatment facilities. While the evaluation process can differ across treatment facilities, most evaluations include many parts described in this chapter. These include interviews, behavioral observations, mental status exams, other records, collateral information, a physical exam, cognitive assessments, lab tests, an EEG, and imaging studies. The goal of an evaluation is to better understand what the patient is experiencing, provide an explanation for the family, give a correct diagnosis, and develop an effective treatment plan with the patient.

Patients, family members, and friends can help the evaluation process by providing important information to mental health professionals. Today, many individuals diagnosed with psychosis are able to achieve a meaningful level of recovery. This would be very unlikely if the individual never came in for an evaluation and treatment. Patients and their family members should not hesitate in seeking treatment. Evaluation is the first step towards recovery.

Key Chapter Points

- ☞ The evaluation process is the first step in helping people who are experiencing a first psychotic episode.
- ☞ The evaluation process can provide families with an explanation for what their loved one is experiencing. It also may help the patient to feel better understood.
- ☞ Although the interview and behavioral observations can be done in inpatient or outpatient settings, treatment of early psychosis often happens in inpatient settings because of symptom severity.
- ☞ Sometimes the evaluation may include gathering additional information from sources other than the patient.
- ☞ Patients often receive a physical exam to look for any physical problems that may have led to the psychosis, as well as lab tests, an EEG, and imaging studies.
- ☞ Understanding the evaluation process and being able to provide mental health professionals with information can help in the evaluation and treatment planning.

Acknowledgment: This chapter was initially developed by Hanan D. Trotman, MA.

6

Medicines Used to Treat Psychosis

Mental health professionals treat nearly all psychiatric illnesses using two types of treatments: medicines and psychosocial treatments. This is true for psychosis as well. We describe medicines used to treat psychosis in this chapter and psychosocial treatments for psychosis in Chapter 7. Medicines are a crucial part of the treatment plan for people who experience a first episode of psychosis. In fact, many mental health professionals view medicines to be the most important aspect of the treatment of psychosis. This is because psychosocial treatments are usually more effective when medicines help to adequately control symptoms.

We discuss a number of medicines in this chapter. When a specific medicine is mentioned, two names are given. The first is the **generic name** and the second (in parentheses) is the **trade name** in the United States. For example, Tylenol is the trade name of the generic pain medicine called acetaminophen. Anyone taking medicine should be familiar with both the generic and trade names of the medicine, even though the generic names are sometimes more difficult to spell or pronounce.

This chapter begins with an overview of the class of medicines used to treat psychosis, called antipsychotic medicines, or just "antipsychotics." Before explaining antipsychotics in further detail, we set the stage by defining (1) how antipsychotics work and (2) some side effects and other serious problems called adverse events that may occur when taking antipsychotics. We then describe in more detail the two main types of medicines used to treat psychosis, the so-called "conventional" antipsychotics, and the "atypical" antipsychotics. Some mental health professionals refer to these as "first-generation" and "second-generation" antipsychotics, respectively. Then, we discuss the sometimes difficult task of finding the right medicine. We end by addressing two commonly asked questions about antipsychotic medicines: "Why is it important to take the medicine?" and "How long should the medicine be taken?"

Antipsychotic Medicines

As mentioned earlier, the main types of medicines used to treat psychosis are the **antipsychotics**. These medicines are "antipsychotics" because they fight against ("anti-") psychotic symptoms. As discussed in Chapter 1 (What Is Psychosis?) and Chapter 2 (What Are the Symptoms of Psychosis?), psychosis is a state of not being well-grounded in reality, due to symptoms like hallucinations or delusions. So, the term *antipsychotic medicines* means that this group of medicines works best for positive symptoms. Researchers are working to develop medicines that will be helpful for the other types of symptoms associated with psychosis, including negative symptoms and cognitive dysfunction.

> The term antipsychotic medicines means that this group of medicines works best for positive symptoms. Researchers are working to develop medicines that will be helpful for the other types of symptoms associated with psychosis, including negative symptoms and cognitive dysfunction.

There are over 60 different antipsychotic medicines in use around the world. About 20 of these are available in the United States, giving mental health professionals many options in choosing a medicine to treat hallucinations and delusions. In general, antipsychotic medicines can be divided into two types, the older ones and the newer ones. The older medicines are referred to using various terms, including: *first-generation antipsychotics*, *conventional antipsychotics*, *typical antipsychotics*, *neuroleptics*, and *major tranquilizers*. In this chapter, we use the phrase **conventional antipsychotics** for the older antipsychotics. The newer medicines are referred to either as *second-generation antipsychotics* or *atypical antipsychotics*. In this chapter, we use the term **atypical antipsychotics** for the newer medicines.

How Do Antipsychotics Work?

When a person swallows a pill or capsule, some portion of the chemical inside the pill or capsule will be absorbed from the digestive system into the bloodstream. For psychiatric medicines, some portion of this absorbed chemical will then enter the brain from the bloodstream. It is in the brain that antipsychotics have their helpful effects. For the few antipsychotics that are available as a long-acting shot given every two to four weeks, the chemical in the shot is slowly absorbed from the muscle into the bloodstream.

Once in the brain, the active ingredient of the medicine binds to **receptors**. Receptors are proteins on the surface of cells, such as nerve cells or neurons. When the chemical binds to the receptor on the surface of a neuron in the brain, the chemical can either "turn on" or "turn off" the receptor. This binding to the receptor protein therefore either mimics the usual actions of natural chemicals within the brain ("turning on") or decreases the usual actions of such chemicals ("turning off").

This binding and "turning on" or "turning off" of the receptor by the medicine then causes further chemical changes that affect the ways that neurons communicate with one another. Nearly all medicines used to treat psychiatric illnesses, including antidepressants, mood stabilizers, anti-anxiety medicines, sleep medicines, and antipsychotics, bind to different types of receptors in brain pathways that regulate mood, anxiety, sleep, thinking, attention, etc.

All currently available antipsychotics bind to dopamine receptors in the brain. Dopamine is a natural chemical in the brain that allows certain neurons to communicate with one another. Dopamine neurons are involved in movements, pleasure and reward, thinking, and senses such as seeing and hearing. Antipsychotics bind to and turn off a certain type of dopamine receptor called the D_2 receptor. Doing this turns down the dopamine communication between neurons, which better regulates these brain pathways in people with psychosis. The well-known fact that antipsychotic medicines turn off dopamine receptors on certain neurons has led scientists to think that part of the cause of schizophrenia may be related to abnormal levels of dopamine in certain parts of the brain (see Chapter 4 on What Causes Primary Psychotic Disorders Like Schizophrenia?).

Research has proven that antipsychotic medicines work. In fact, doctors think that all patients with psychosis should take an antipsychotic medicine, just as all people with pneumonia due to bacteria should take an antibiotic. That is, they are helpful in decreasing or getting rid of symptoms, such as hallucinations like hearing voices. They are also helpful in decreasing one's focus on delusions, or gradually removing delusions altogether. They treat a number of other symptoms, such as paranoia, as well. They are somewhat helpful for other types of symptoms, though further research is required to develop better medicines to treat negative symptoms and cognitive dysfunction associated with psychosis.

> Research has proven that antipsychotic medicines work. In fact, doctors think that all patients with psychosis should take an antipsychotic medicine, just as all people with pneumonia due to bacteria should take an antibiotic.

What Are Side Effects?

Unfortunately, some antipsychotics bind to other types of receptors in the brain, such as **acetylcholine**, **histamine**, and **norepinephrine** receptors, and this can be the cause of some of the **side effects** of antipsychotics. Side effects are unwanted effects of medicines. For example, an antipsychotic medicine that binds to and turns down acetylcholine receptors in addition to dopamine receptors may cause a dry mouth. Binding to and turning down histamine receptors may lead to sleepiness, and binding to and turning down norepinephrine may lead to changes in blood pressure. Descriptions of side effects that may happen when taking specific antipsychotics follow in the sections on Conventional Antipsychotics and Atypical Antipsychotics.

All medicines can cause side effects, but not every person taking a particular medicine will have side effects. In fact, most people do not experience side effects from their medicines. Table 6.1 lists some of the side effects that may occur when taking an antipsychotic

Table 6.1 Common Side Effects that May Occur When Taking an Antipsychotic Medicine

- General Side Effects
  - ° Blurry vision
  - ° Constipation
  - ° Dry mouth
  - ° Headache
  - ° Insomnia (difficulty falling asleep or staying asleep)
  - ° Sexual side effects (such as decreased sex drive)
  - ° Sleepiness/sedation/drowsiness
  - ° Upset stomach (nausea, vomiting, diarrhea)
- Secondary Negative Symptoms
  - ° Decreased creativity
  - ° Decreased emotion
  - ° Feeling cloudy or foggy
  - ° Slowness
- Extrapyramidal Side Effects (see Table 6.3)
- Metabolic Side Effects (see Table 6.5)
- Side Effects from Elevated Prolactin Levels
  - ° Menstrual irregularities in women
  - ° Breast enlargement, breast tenderness, or milk production in women
  - ° Growth of breast tissue in men
  - ° Weight gain

medicine. It is important to discuss possible side effects from specific medicines with the psychiatrist. That way, patients and families will know which particular side effects to look out for and how to handle them if they do occur.

Side effects are most likely to occur when a medicine is just being started, and side effects often go away after several days or weeks of taking the medicine. Mental health professionals are very interested in hearing from patients about whether or not they are having any side effects. Mental health professionals want to work closely with patients to find the right dose of medicine that works the best, while at the same time minimizing side effects as much as possible.

When a patient has a side effect, the doctor has several options to try to decrease the side effect. Some of these options are listed below:

- If it is likely that the side effect will go away after a few days or weeks, the doctor may ask the patient to try to continue taking the medicine despite having a side effect.

- The doctor may carefully decrease the dose of the medicine a little to try to remove the side effect while keeping the helpful effects.
- The doctor may change the way the patient takes the medicine, such as dividing the dose and taking it twice a day (once in the morning and once at night) instead of once a day.
- The doctor may start another medicine to try to decrease the side effect.
- The patient may need to switch to another medicine that hopefully will not cause the side effect (see the following pages for ways that doctors switch medicines).

What Are Adverse Events?

Adverse events are similar to side effects in that they are unwanted effects of medicines. As noted earlier, side effects are relatively common, often happen when the patient first starts taking the medicine, and often go away with some time. However, adverse events are much rarer, may happen at any time when taking the medicine (not just when starting the medicine or increasing the dose), and sometimes may not go away. Also, whereas side effects are usually mild and often can be tolerated, adverse events are serious and at times may even be life-threatening.

Just as all medicines used by doctors to treat any disease can cause some side effects, many medicines can also cause these rare adverse events. Examples of an adverse event are an allergic reaction to penicillin, fainting caused by a blood pressure medicine, swelling of the tongue caused by a blood pressure medicine, bleeding in the stomach caused by a pain medicine, or extremely low blood sugar caused by insulin. These are all serious and require immediate medical attention. Antipsychotic medicines do not cause most of these adverse events, but they can cause other adverse events in rare instances. We describe rare adverse events that may happen when taking specific antipsychotics in later sections of this chapter. When a patient has an adverse event, the doctor often will switch the medicine immediately. Other options may include decreasing the dose, adding another medicine to treat the adverse event, or gradually switching to a different medicine (again, see the following pages for ways that doctors switch medicines).

Conventional Antipsychotics

As mentioned earlier, there are two types of antipsychotic medicines: conventional antipsychotics (the older ones) and atypical antipsychotics (the newer ones). The conventional antipsychotics were first discovered in the 1950s. Before that time, there were almost no treatments for psychosis in the form of medicines. In the 1950s through the 1980s, a number of conventional antipsychotics were developed. Table 6.2 lists some of these, though there are more than 50 such conventional antipsychotics in use around the world. The conventional antipsychotics are proven to be helpful in reducing the symptoms of psychosis, especially hallucinations, delusions, paranoia, and disorganized thinking. They are less effective in treating some of the other types of symptoms, including negative symptoms and cognitive dysfunction.

Some of the side effects that may happen when taking conventional antipsychotics include blurry vision, constipation, dizziness upon standing, dry mouth, sleepiness, low blood pressure, and upset stomach. Conventional antipsychotics can also cause a dulling or slowing of thinking and movements that is referred to as "secondary negative symptoms" because they mimic the negative symptoms of schizophrenia, but they come from the medicine.

A common set of side effects of conventional antipsychotics are the **extrapyramidal side effects (EPS)**. EPS are a number of movement side effects, which we list and define in Table 6.3. EPS can be quite common when taking conventional antipsychotics. They are much less likely to occur when taking the newer atypical antipsychotic medicines

Table 6.2 Some of the Many Conventional Antipsychotic Medicines

- chlorpromazine (Thorazine)
- fluphenazine (Prolixin)
- haloperidol (Haldol)
- loxapine (Loxitane)
- mesoridazine (Serentil)
- molindone (Moban)
- perphenazine (Trilafon)
- pimozide (Orap)
- thioridazine (Mellaril)
- thiothixene (Navane)
- trifluoperazine (Stelazine)

Table 6.3 The Various Forms of Extrapyramidal Side Effects (EPS)
of Antipsychotic Medicines

Type of EPS	Description	Appearance
Acute dystonia	This side effect usually comes on suddenly. It typically involves painful tightening of a muscle or muscle group.	* Oculogyric crisis: sudden, painful tightening of the eye muscles * Torticollis: sudden, painful neck spasm * Dystonia: the sudden, painful contraction of a muscle or muscle group
Akathisia	An inner sense of restlessness, fidgetiness, or inner need to move	* Anxiety * Fidgeting * Pacing * Constant shifting or moving of legs
Parkinsonism	A group of side effects that mimic the symptoms of Parkinson's disease	* Decreased facial expression * Fine tremor of the hands * Handwriting becomes very small * Slow, shuffling gait * Slowing of movements * Stiffness of muscles

described next. Oftentimes, EPS are treated by adding another medicine that is used specifically to treat the EPS. Such medicines may include benztropine (Cogentin), diphenhydramine (Benadryl), hydroxyzine (Atarax, Vistaril), or trihexyphenidyl (Artane).

Another side effect that may happen when taking conventional antipsychotics is an elevation in the **prolactin** level in the blood. Prolactin is a hormone secreted by the pituitary gland in the brain. Confirming an elevated prolactin level requires drawing a sample of blood to be sent to the lab. An increase in the prolactin level can cause a number of side effects. For example, in women, an increase in the prolactin level can cause breast enlargement or tenderness, and even milk production despite not being pregnant. It can also cause the menstrual cycle to become irregular or to stop. In men, an elevated prolactin level can cause the breast tissue to grow. In both men and women, an elevated prolactin level also can be one cause of weight gain. If the prolactin elevation is mild, it may not cause any side effects and may not require treatment. However, if the elevation of prolactin level in the blood causes side effects, the doctor will often decrease the dose of the antipsychotic or will add another medicine to reduce the prolactin level. Although an elevated prolactin level is usually an issue only with the conventional antipsychotics, one of the newer atypical antipsychotics described in the following pages, risperidone (Risperdal), also may cause elevated prolactin levels.

Several adverse events may happen when taking conventional antipsychotics. Rarely, these medicines can cause an allergic reaction, such as hives and itching, a swollen airway or tongue, or difficulty breathing. Conventional antipsychotics can sometimes cause a seizure, especially in people who have a tendency to have seizures or who are taking another medicine that also can cause seizures. Very rarely, such medicines may cause dysfunction of specific organs, like the liver (hepatitis) or the pancreas (pancreatitis).

One important adverse event that is much more common with conventional antipsychotics than with atypical antipsychotics is **tardive dyskinesia (TD)**. TD is an adverse event that develops after extended periods (months, years, or decades) of taking conventional antipsychotics. TD consists of abnormal, involuntary movements. These movements often involve the mouth (chewing or puckering movements), the fingers or toes, or the trunk (such as rocking or swaying). When using conventional antipsychotics, doctors often assess for TD regularly, such as every six months, by carefully observing the tongue, fingers, and toes for abnormal, involuntary movements.

Despite the possibility of having side effects or rare adverse events, conventional antipsychotics are very helpful in treating psychosis in many people. In fact, for some people, these older medicines seem to be even more helpful than the newer medicines. However, nowadays most patients with a first episode of psychosis are initially treated with one of the newer medicines, an atypical antipsychotic.

Atypical Antipsychotics

Only conventional antipsychotics were available from the mid to late 1950s through the early 1990s. Beginning in the 1990s, a newer class of antipsychotics was developed. In addition to binding to and turning off dopamine receptors, these newer medicines also bind to certain **serotonin** receptors. Serotonin is another natural chemical in the brain that appears to play a role in the mental functions affected by psychosis.

You may be wondering why mental health professionals call the newer antipsychotics "atypical." There are several ways in which the newer medicines differ from conventional antipsychotics, leading mental health professionals to call the newer, second-generation antipsychotics "atypical." Some of the reasons for this terminology are:

- The beneficial effects of these medicines appear to be related to the fact that they bind to serotonin receptors in addition to dopamine receptors.
- These medicines may be more helpful in treating certain types of symptoms, like negative symptoms and cognitive dysfunction, compared to the older, conventional medicines.
- These medicines are generally less likely to cause EPS.
- Most of these medicines are less likely to cause elevated prolactin levels.
- Perhaps most importantly, these medicines are less likely to cause TD, even after taking them for years.

Like the conventional antipsychotics, atypical antipsychotics have been proven to be helpful in reducing the symptoms of psychosis, especially hallucinations, delusions, paranoia, and disorganized thinking. Some doctors and researchers believe that atypical antipsychotics may be somewhat more effective in treating some of the other types of symptoms, like negative symptoms and cognitive dysfunction. More than 10 atypical antipsychotics are in use around the world, and several of these are listed, along with the usual daily starting dose and typical effective dose, in Table 6.4.

Many mental health professionals view atypical antipsychotics as the first-choice medicines for the treatment of psychosis. So, doctors often prefer to use these newer agents first, reserving the older medicines for use only if atypical antipsychotics prove unsuccessful.

Table 6.4 Atypical Antipsychotic Medicines Currently Available in the United States

Generic Name (Trade Name)	Usual Daily Starting Dose	Typical Daily Effective Dose
clozapine (Clozaril)	25 mg	400–600 mg
risperidone (Risperdal)	1–2 mg	2–6 mg
olanzapine (Zyprexa)	5–10 mg	10–30 mg
quetiapine (Seroquel)	100–200 mg	300–800 mg
ziprasidone (Geodon)	40–80 mg	120–240 mg
aripiprazole (Abilify)	5–15 mg	10–30 mg
paliperidone (Invega)	3–6 mg	3–12 mg

Unfortunately, the atypical antipsychotics are generally much more expensive than the conventional antipsychotics.

Researchers have studied the effects of atypical antipsychotics on other psychiatric illnesses, in addition to psychosis. Government agencies (like the Food and Drug Administration (FDA), in the United States) have approved some of these medicines for the treatment of bipolar disorder, major depression, dementia, and other disorders in addition to psychosis.

Some of the side effects that may happen when taking atypical antipsychotics include the same side effects that may occur when taking conventional antipsychotics: blurry vision, constipation, dizziness upon standing, dry mouth, sleepiness, low blood pressure, and upset stomach. As noted earlier, most atypical antipsychotics are less likely to cause EPS and elevated prolactin levels. In general, atypical antipsychotics are usually well tolerated by patients, meaning that they usually do not cause excessive side effects. This is especially true when these medicines are used at relatively low doses, which is often the case for patients going through the initial evaluation and treatment of new-onset psychosis.

Two important types of side effects that occur when taking some of the atypical antipsychotics are **weight gain** and **metabolic side effects**. These side effects are especially likely to occur with clozapine (Clozaril) and olanzapine (Zyprexa), but nearly any antipsychotic medicine may stimulate appetite and cause weight gain. Because of the possibility of these side effects, doctors prescribing atypical antipsychotics closely monitor the patient's weight and periodically check certain labs, like **fasting glucose and lipids** (see Table 6.5). This requires drawing a sample of blood to be sent to the lab. Careful monitoring for weight gain and metabolic side effects is crucial because both have negative long-term health consequences. If the doctor sees that such side effects are developing, he or she may try one or more of the strategies listed earlier to decrease the side effects.

One of the atypical antipsychotics, called clozapine (Clozaril), can cause several serious adverse events. These include agranulocytosis (a sudden and dangerous drop in the white blood cell count that leaves the person susceptible to severe infections), myocarditis (an inflammation of the heart muscle), and seizures. Because of the rare risk of agranulocytosis, patients taking clozapine must have weekly (or biweekly)

Table 6.5 Weight Gain and Metabolic Side Effects that May Be
Caused by Atypical Antipsychotic Medicines and Ways that
Doctors Monitor for These Side Effects

Side Effects	Ways to Monitor
Weight Gain	Waist circumference, body weight
Metabolic Side Effects Elevated triglycerides Elevated low-density lipoprotein (LDL) cholesterol Low high-density lipoprotein (HDL) cholesterol Elevated glucose (sugar)	Blood samples for fasting lipids (triglycerides and cholesterol) and fasting glucose

blood draws to closely monitor the white blood cell count. This is necessary even though the risk of agranulocytosis is only about 1%.

The risk of these adverse events with clozapine is particularly unfortunate because, of all of the antipsychotics, clozapine appears to be the one that is most helpful in treating psychosis that does not respond to other antipsychotics. In fact, clozapine is often reserved for patients with **treatment-refractory psychosis**, meaning that the psychotic symptoms have not cleared up even after trying several different antipsychotic medicines. Clozapine is more helpful than other medicines for treatment-refractory psychosis.

Finding the Right Antipsychotic Medicine

Research shows that atypical antipsychotics may be somewhat more effective than conventional antipsychotics. This is because they may treat a wider range of symptoms, though this is not always the case. However, all of the atypical antipsychotics appear to be about equally effective (except for the fact that clozapine appears to be more effective than other medicines when psychosis continues despite using other medicines). So, doctors select from among the various antipsychotic medicines based on a number of other factors. These may include:

- whether or not the medicine helped in the past
- the specific symptoms present
- past side effects or expected side effects
- how easy it is to take the medicine (for example, once rather than twice daily)

- the cost of the medicine
- the doctor's own familiarity with specific medicines
- whether or not a family member ever benefited from the medicine

Doctors usually consider all of these factors when working with patients and their families to select a medicine. A simpler way of looking at this is that the doctor is trying to balance the good and bad aspects of the medicine. Namely, he or she wants to maximize the benefits in terms of symptom response, while minimizing side effects and adverse events.

Sometimes the first medicine that is tried is successful. Other times, the first medicine may cause side effects or may not work. In these cases, the doctor may need to switch to another medicine. Usually after one to three different medicines are tried, the best medicine can be identified.

In other cases, if psychotic symptoms are severe, the doctor may want to try a higher dose or increase the dose more rapidly. Related to the balancing work illustrated in Figure 6.1, doctors usually try to find the lowest effective dose in order to minimize side effects. The symptoms of young people with first-episode psychosis often clear up fairly well with a relatively low dose of the antipsychotic. First-episode patients also may be more likely to develop side effects than older patients who have been on medicines longer. For these reasons, doctors often try to find the lowest does that is still effective. However, a dose that is too low may not provide all of the benefits that could be seen with a higher dose. So, doctors work to find an "adequate dose" or a "therapeutic dose" without using more medicine than is necessary.

If the doctor recommends that the medicine be switched to another one (perhaps because of side effects or because of inadequate

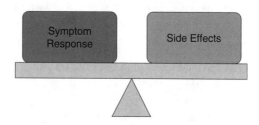

Figure 6.1 Balancing the Benefits and Risks of Antipsychotic Medicines

response), the doctor will decide among several ways how the switch can be made. The switch must be made carefully because any time an antipsychotic medicine is being stopped there is a risk for a relapse of psychotic symptoms. Three methods for making a switch to another medicine include:

- The doctor may stop the first medicine and start the second one.
- The doctor may gradually decrease, or "taper," the first medicine while the second one is being increased, or "titrated" over several days or weeks.
- The doctor may add and increase the second medicine over several days or weeks until it is at an effective dose and then taper or stop the first medicine.

Some patients have a hard time consistently taking their medicine. For these patients, or for those who would rather simply take a shot than a daily pill, several antipsychotic medicines are available as a shot that is given every two to four weeks. Specifically, several conventional antipsychotics are available as a shot, including haloperidol (Haldol) decanoate and fluphenazine (Prolixin) decanoate. Among the atypical antipsychotics, risperidone is available as a long-acting injectable (Risperdal Consta), and others are likely to be developed in upcoming years. These injectable medicines ensure that a steady dose of the drug is delivered to the brain while avoiding the problem of forgetting to take pills once or twice a day.

Several atypical antipsychotics are also available as a special rapidly dissolving tablet, in addition to the regular types of pills or capsules. These special tablets dissolve rapidly (within seconds) when placed in the mouth. With these, the patient does not have to swallow a pill. Such tablets also dissolve before the pill can be spit out.

Other Medicines Sometimes Used in the Treatment of Psychotic Disorders

Sometimes it is necessary to use other types of medicines, in addition to antipsychotics, to target other types of symptoms. For example, antidepressants may be helpful if symptoms of depression are present. Mood stabilizers may be useful if irritability, impulsiveness, hostility, or unstable moods happen. **Anxiety medicines** or **sleep medicines** may be needed if anxiety symptoms or difficulty sleeping are a problem. As mentioned earlier, sometimes medicines used to treat the side effects of antipsychotics, like EPS, may be needed to make it easier to take the antipsychotic medicine. Nearly all of these other medicines are given as a pill or capsule taken orally. Like any other medicine, these medicines also may cause some side effects in some people.

Possible Future Treatments for Psychotic Disorders

Many researchers around the world are working to discover new medicines that will be even more helpful in treating psychosis. Some of the new medicines that will become available in the upcoming years are very different from the conventional antipsychotics and the atypical antipsychotics. They will work in different ways, beyond binding to dopamine or serotonin receptors. Additionally, they will treat a broader range of the symptoms of psychosis. Whereas currently available antipsychotic medicines mainly treat the positive symptoms (like hallucinations and delusions), medicines being developed also will treat negative symptoms and cognitive dysfunction. This is very important research because, as discussed in Chapter 2, negative symptoms and cognitive dysfunction lead to a lot of the disability associated with schizophrenia and other psychotic disorders.

Why Is It Important to Take the Medicine?

Extensive scientific research has proven that antipsychotic medicines, both conventional and atypical antipsychotics, are effective in reducing the symptoms of psychosis. They are especially helpful in decreasing the positive symptoms, such as auditory hallucinations, delusions, paranoia, and ideas of reference. They are also helpful for disorganized thinking. Antipsychotics may help some with negative symptoms and cognitive dysfunction. As noted earlier, ongoing research aims to find even better medicines for psychosis, especially medicines that will be more helpful for negative symptoms and cognitive dysfunction.

Also as noted earlier, many doctors would say that antipsychotic medicines are the most important first step in the treatment of psychosis. By improving the symptoms, patients are better able to follow through with psychosocial treatments (see Chapter 7) designed to promote recovery (see Chapter 11). It is very important that patients take medicines regularly, exactly as prescribed. Sticking with their treatment plan is essential to getting better (see Chapter 8).

The benefits of taking antipsychotic medicines can be thought of in terms of short-term benefits and long-term benefits. The main short-term benefit is the reduction in psychotic symptoms. The long-term benefits of taking antipsychotic medicines stem from this reduction in psychotic symptoms. That is, symptoms are much more likely to clear up when taking antipsychotic medicines. But more importantly, the reduction in psychotic symptoms allows people who have had a psychotic episode to more easily reach their personal goals in areas such as school, work, relationships, and recreation/leisure. In addition to reducing symptoms and promoting recovery, another long-term benefit of taking antipsychotic medicines is that they reduce the chances of a relapse of psychotic symptoms or hospitalization (see Figure 6.2). So, in addition to treating psychotic symptoms in the present, antipsychotic medicines have an important role in relapse prevention for the future.

> In addition to reducing symptoms and promoting recovery, another long-term benefit of taking antipsychotic medicines is that they reduce the chances of a relapse of psychotic symptoms or hospitalization. So, in addition to treating psychotic symptoms in the present, antipsychotic medicines have an important role in relapse prevention for the future.

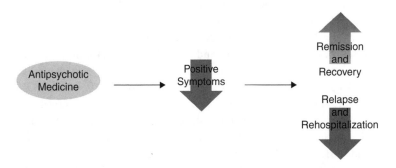

Figure 6.2 The Short-term and Long-term Benefits of Antipsychotic Medicines

How Long Should the Medicine Be Taken?

The first step in the process of taking an antipsychotic medicine is the initial stabilization. Here, the goal is to get rid of the positive symptoms (**remission**). Approximately 85% of patients with new-onset or first-episode psychosis are able to achieve symptom remission over the course of about three months. In many cases, remission may occur even sooner. In general, hallucinations, like hearing voices, may get much better or go away after several days to several weeks on the medicine. Delusions and disorganized thinking often take longer, often several weeks to several months, to get better or go away. This is another reason why it is crucial to stay on the medicine—so that the full effects can be seen over time.

Doctors want to work closely with patients to decide how long they should take medicines. In some cases, it is clear to the doctor, based on the types of symptoms present, that the medicine should be continued long-term, perhaps even lifelong. In other cases, if symptoms seem to resolve completely, the doctor may recommend a very gradual and careful reduction of the dose. This would usually only happen after complete remission of symptoms for at least six months to two years.

Some patients eventually may be able to stop taking the medicine. This is done very carefully with the patient's mental health professionals and the patient working together. Instead of stopping suddenly, the medicine may be gradually decreased over several months. Patients, their families, and their mental health professionals must watch for any return of symptoms or early warning signs (see Chapter 9). However, most patients who have had a psychotic episode and receive a diagnosis of a psychotic disorder like schizophrenia will need to continue the medicine long-term.

People who experience a first episode of psychosis should not stop their medicines suddenly and should not decrease or stop their medicines without working closely with the doctor. Any change in the dose of the medicine needs very close monitoring. Sometimes this close monitoring may require drawing a blood sample to check the level of the medicine in the bloodstream. This may help the doctor to decide if the dose is right. Fortunately, antipsychotic medicines are not addictive or habit-forming.

Recent research suggests that one of the biggest problems in the treatment of psychosis is that many patients stop their medicine on their own. For example, some studies show that approximately 70% of patients being treated in the early course of a psychotic disorder stop taking the medicine within one year. Common reasons for stopping the medicine may be because it is not working well enough, because of side effects, or because the patient simply decides to stop taking it for other reasons (often due to impaired insight or other types of symptoms). Also, substance abuse can interfere with the patient's ability to continue taking the medicine as prescribed. Stopping the medicine is problematic because it greatly increases the chance of relapse of symptoms, often requiring hospitalization. Furthermore, stopping the medicine commonly interferes with a person's ability to continue pursuing his or her goals for recovery. For these reasons, mental health professionals usually strongly encourage patients with a psychotic disorder to follow the medicine plan exactly as prescribed (see Chapter 8). If the patient does stop taking the medicine, the doctor will want to continue seeing the patient and providing support in other ways, such as counseling and psychoeducation.

Putting It All Together

Both conventional and atypical antipsychotic medicines are helpful in reducing psychotic symptoms. These medicines work by blocking and therefore "turning off" certain types of receptors on neurons in the brain, such as dopamine and serotonin receptors. Side effects may occur with any medicine, including antipsychotic medicines. Different antipsychotic medicines have different types of possible side effects and adverse events. For example, whereas conventional antipsychotics can cause extrapyramidal side effects (EPS), elevated prolactin levels, or tardive dyskinesia (TD), the newer atypical antipsychotics may cause weight gain and metabolic side effects in some people.

Because antipsychotics are proven to be effective in reducing psychotic symptoms, and because side effects may happen, doctors work closely with patients and their families to balance the benefits and risks and find the right medicine for each patient experiencing psychosis. Mental health professionals recommend that the medicine be continued as prescribed to improve one's likelihood of remission. This in turn provides longer-term benefits by promoting recovery and preventing relapse.

Worksheet 6.1 Medicines Prescribed

The amount of information that you have to keep track of can be overwhelming at times. Here is a place to mark the type of medicines included in the treatment plan. It also is a place to keep instructions for taking those medicines.

Name of Medicine	Dose	How Often/When to Take Medicine	Special Instructions from the Doctor

Key Chapter Points

- ☛ Many mental health professionals view medicines to be the most important aspect of the treatment of psychosis.
- ☛ The main types of medicines used to treat psychosis are antipsychotics, named this because this group of medicines is most effective for positive symptoms.
- ☛ Antipsychotics work by binding to dopamine receptors in the brain, which affects the ways certain chemicals communicate with each other.
- ☛ There are two types of antipsychotics, conventional antipsychotics (the older ones) and atypical antipsychotics (the newer ones).
- ☛ Sometimes antipsychotics cause side effects. It is important to discuss possible side effects from specific medicines with the psychiatrist, so that patients and families know which side effects to expect and how to handle these if they happen.
- ☛ When prescribing medicines, doctors try to balance the good and bad aspects of the medicine to maximize the benefits in terms of symptom response, while minimizing side effects and adverse events.
- ☛ Research has proven that antipsychotics are effective in reducing symptoms, especially positive symptoms. By improving symptoms, patients are better able to follow through with psychosocial treatments designed to promote recovery.
- ☛ The length of time that the medicine should be taken is based on the types of symptoms the patient experiences and how long the symptoms last.

7

Psychosocial Treatments for Early Psychosis

People experiencing psychosis often have to deal with a number of problems. These problems may stem from certain symptoms. As explained in Chapter 2, these symptoms may include positive symptoms (such as hearing voices or having unusual beliefs), negative symptoms (such as being isolated, withdrawn, or slow), cognitive dysfunction (such as difficulties with attention, learning, or memory), and other types of symptoms. However, psychosocial difficulties (like problems with school, work, relationships, and recreation/leisure activities) may disrupt life as well, even though they are not necessarily thought of as symptoms.

Unfortunately, these types of problems are very common for people dealing with a psychotic disorder. Treating these difficulties in addition to the specific symptoms is necessary to begin to feel better and to live a full life. In fact, the recovery process focuses as much on resuming school, work, relationships, and leisure activities as it does on remission (see Chapter 11 on Promoting Recovery). Although medicines are extremely important in treating symptoms, especially positive symptoms (see Chapter 6 on Medicines Used to Treat Psychosis), another type of treatments, called **psychosocial treatments,** focus more on helping patients with these broader problems.

Psychosocial Problems Caused by Psychosis

Normal **psychosocial development** begins in childhood but continues throughout adolescence and early adulthood. Adolescence and early adulthood are extremely important times when most people develop social skills and build relationships. Late adolescence and early adulthood is typically a time of finishing high school, starting college, getting a first job, having a first romantic relationship, beginning to live more independently from parents, buying a car, and establishing career goals. Success in all of these domains of life requires both psychological skills and social skills. The term *psychosocial* brings together these two words. So, psychosocial development refers to the important developmental stage when psychological and social skills mature.

Unfortunately, for people who develop a psychotic disorder, late adolescence and early adulthood is the period of time when a first episode of psychosis usually begins. Thus, psychosis that first happens in this time period often interrupts psychosocial development, leading to psychosocial problems.

> Unfortunately, for people who develop a psychotic disorder, late adolescence and early adulthood is the period of time when a first episode of psychosis usually begins. Thus, psychosis that first happens in this time period often interrupts psychosocial development, leading to psychosocial problems.

Psychosocial problems refer to difficulties at school, at work, in relationships, or in recreation and leisure activities. Psychosocial problems may come about when someone does not have the skills needed to successfully interact with his or her social environment. Some psychosocial problems that are common among people experiencing an episode of psychosis include the following:

- declining grades
- dropping out of school
- difficulty getting along with coworkers
- losing a job
- not having friends
- conflicts within the family

- conflicts within a relationship
- trouble maintaining housing
- not maintaining personal hygiene
- giving up hobbies
- having no leisure activities

Psychosocial Treatments

As described earlier, individuals experiencing a psychotic episode in late adolescence or early adulthood typically face an interruption in normal psychosocial development. The purpose of psychosocial treatments is to help patients with psychosis or other serious mental illnesses to overcome psychosocial problems and to resume psychosocial development. Psychosocial treatments attempt to change behaviors by focusing on problems patients have interacting with their social environments. Mental health professionals sometimes use the word **psychosocial rehabilitation** to describe many psychosocial treatments. This means that treatment increases psychosocial skills to the best possible level of functioning. In other words, psychosocial rehabilitation aims to reduce the problems patients experience and to maximize abilities in areas such as school, work, relationship, and recreation/leisure.

There are several types of psychosocial treatments. In some cases, mental health professionals recommend several different psychosocial treatments at once. These treatments are always given in combination with a medicine. Without the use of a medicine to treat key symptoms, many psychosocial treatments would be unsuccessful. However, just as medicines can improve success in psychosocial treatments, psychosocial treatments (like cognitive-behavioral therapy, psychoeducation, and family psychoeducation) can improve patients' success in medicine treatment. This is because they may improve adherence with the medicine.

While the main purpose of medicine is to lessen the severity of symptoms such as hallucinations, psychosocial treatments focus on other areas of life affected by psychosis such as school and work functioning, relationships, and quality of life. In this way, medicine and psychosocial treatments complement each other as they both target different aspects of the illness.

While the main purpose of medicine is to lessen the severity of symptoms such as hallucinations, psychosocial treatments focus on other areas of life affected by psychosis such as school and work functioning, relationships, and quality of life. In this way, medicine and psychosocial treatments complement each other as they both target different aspects of the illness.

The Need for Some Level of Reality Testing and Insight

Psychosocial treatments can be most successful when the patient has (1) an adequate level of reality testing, and (2) some insight into his or her problems. **Reality testing** refers to one's ability to decide between what is real and what is not real. Because psychosis refers to a mental state of being out of touch with reality, someone who is psychotic has an impairment in reality testing (for example, hearing voices or having unusual beliefs). Before psychosocial treatments can be effective, psychosis usually needs to be somewhat under control. For example, knowing when the auditory hallucinations are not really coming from another person or being able to understand that delusional ideas may not represent true reality is an important step towards reality testing. A certain level of reality testing can help people with a psychotic disorder engage in psychosocial treatments.

As described in Chapter 2, **impaired insight** is often a major problem for patients with psychosis. Impaired insight is usually related to the illness itself and the nature of the symptoms, not due to a denial or refusal to try to understand. Unfortunately, nearly all people with psychosis have some level of impaired insight. This lack of insight negatively affects treatment. The patient usually needs to have some level of insight before psychosocial treatments can be effective. For example, understanding that medicines can improve symptoms caused by the illness is an important step towards gaining insight. Mental health professionals work to increase the patient's understanding of the illness, or insight, so that psychosocial treatments can be more effective.

Although it is generally true that an adequate level of reality testing and some insight make psychosocial treatments easier, reality testing and insight are not absolutely necessary for all psychosocial interventions. For example, in cognitive-behavioral therapy (described later in this chapter), the basis for a successful therapy is often good **rapport** (a good working relationship with the therapist), which then allows two different versions of reality to be tested against each other. It is at this point that attitudes about and beliefs in delusions or hallucinations may begin to shift. Rapport and trust are often more important to begin with than the level of insight of the person with psychosis

Starting and Sticking with Psychosocial Treatments

Many patients and their families are scared to begin treatment because they do not know what to expect. However, getting help as early as possible will lead to the best results. After an initial thorough evaluation for psychosis (see Chapter 5), the mental health professional doing the evaluation may recommend one or more psychosocial treatments in addition to medicine. The first step in beginning a psychosocial treatment, if the mental health professional doing the initial evaluation is not able to provide it himself or herself, is the referral process. A **referral** is when a health-care professional recommends that a patient goes to a particular type of treatment. For example, a primary care doctor treating a patient with diabetes may give the patient a referral to meet with a dietary counselor or nutritionist. Similarly, a psychiatrist treating a patient with a psychotic episode may give him or her a referral to a psychosocial treatment program. After the doctor gives a referral, the next step is to keep the appointment with the professional specializing in the psychosocial treatment.

Psychosocial treatments often last from six weeks to six months. However, sometimes psychosocial treatments can last for longer periods. For example, residential programs where people live (such as supportive housing), assertive community treatment (described later in the chapter), or day treatment programs may be longer-term. The time in treatment depends on the needs of the particular person with psychosis. We discuss the importance of sticking with treatment in Chapter 8.

A number of different psychosocial treatments are useful for many different mental illnesses, not just psychosis. Psychosocial treatments may be available in a number of treatment settings, including hospitals, mental health clinics, and private offices of mental health professionals. Some psychosocial treatments are available in programs that focus specifically on young people with a first episode of psychosis. We discuss these specialized clinics in Chapter 14.

Psychosocial treatment plans may consist of a single psychosocial treatment. But in some cases, combining several psychosocial treatments may be more effective because they allow patients and their families to begin working on several types of problems at once. We describe nine different types of psychosocial treatments in the following pages and summarize them in Figure 7.1.

Cognitive-Behavioral Therapy

Mental health professionals provide a number of different types of counseling, or psychotherapy, for a variety of mental illnesses. One type of counseling sometimes used for people experiencing an episode of psychosis is **cognitive-behavioral therapy (CBT)**. CBT targets the specific thoughts and beliefs that an individual has that make symptoms worse. It assumes that one's thoughts affect both feelings and behaviors.

What does this mean that one's "thoughts affect both feelings and behaviors"? Here's an example. A teen-aged boy, named Aaron was not picked for the school football team and felt bad. He then did not want to talk to his friend Tim, who had been picked for the team. A CBT approach may help Aaron realize that not being picked for the team made him think to himself that he was a loser. The thought that he was a loser then made him feel sad. He also thought he must be a worse player than his friend Tim, and so he did not speak to Tim when he saw him. Thus, Aaron's thought (that he was a "loser"), which may not have been completely accurate, affected both his feelings (causing him to feel sad) and his behaviors (causing him to avoid talking to his friend Tim.)

CBT is a commonly used form of psychotherapy that is helpful for a variety of mental illnesses including depression, anxiety, and eating disorders. In the case of depression, CBT may help patients to stop thinking of negative things that make them feel down and depressed. For individuals with psychosis, CBT helps patients to consider other explanations for symptoms like delusional ideas, paranoia, and hearing voices. The therapist encourages patients to challenge their

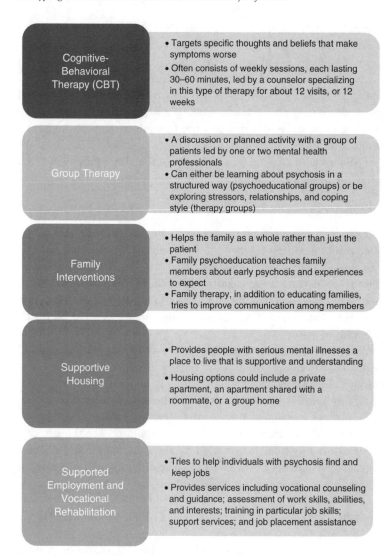

Figure 7.1 Types of Psychosocial Treatments

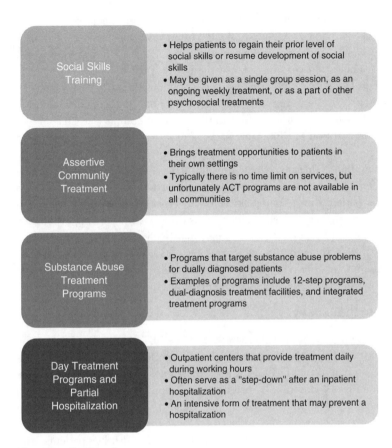

Social Skills Training
- Helps patients to regain their prior level of social skills or resume development of social skills
- May be given as a single group session, as an ongoing weekly treatment, or as a part of other psychosocial treatments

Assertive Community Treatment
- Brings treatment opportunities to patients in their own settings
- Typically there is no time limit on services, but unfortunately ACT programs are not available in all communities

Substance Abuse Treatment Programs
- Programs that target substance abuse problems for dually diagnosed patients
- Examples of programs include 12-step programs, dual-diagnosis treatment facilities, and integrated treatment programs

Day Treatment Programs and Partial Hospitalization
- Outpatient centers that provide treatment daily during working hours
- Often serve as a "step-down" after an inpatient hospitalization
- An intensive form of treatment that may prevent a hospitalization

Figure 7.1 Continued

delusions. As a result, patients learn to do behavioral experiments to test their belief system. Similarly, patients can test and challenge auditory hallucinations so that they come to recognize them as symptoms produced by their brain. Through CBT, patients can also learn helpful coping strategies and rational responses to symptoms. Patients learn useful skills and strategies, such as distraction techniques. CBT may also be helpful in targeting and improving negative symptoms.

Mental health professionals use CBT along with medicine, not as a replacement for medicine. CBT often consists of weekly sessions, each lasting 30–60 minutes, led by a counselor specializing in this type of therapy. A course of CBT often lasts for about 12 visits, or 12 weeks. However, it may be shorter or longer. After therapy ends, patients often continue to use the skills learned in CBT to manage their symptoms. CBT can also help patients to identify early signs of a relapse. Recognizing early warning signs helps patients to act quickly at the earliest sign of a return of psychotic symptoms (see Chapter 9).

In addition to CBT, some patients with psychosis may benefit from other forms of individual therapy or counseling. These may include **compliance therapy**, which aims to increase a patient's abilities to regularly take medicine, or **supportive psychotherapy**, which supports the patient's best coping skills. Other types of individual counseling or therapy may focus on unconscious drives behind feelings, thoughts, and behaviors, or the patient's personality characteristics. In addition, **cognitive remediation**, which may use games and exercises, may be helpful in improving cognitive dysfunction, including difficulties in attention, learning, memory, and planning.

Group Therapy

While individual psychotherapy, such as CBT, takes place one-on-one between the patient and a mental health professional, **group therapy** is when one or two mental health professionals lead a group of patients in a discussion or a planned activity. Group therapy may be available in an inpatient (hospital) or outpatient (clinic) treatment setting. Group therapy allows patients to learn not only from the therapist, but also from the interactions between the therapist and other patients, and other patients and themselves. This form of psychosocial treatment also can help patients to feel less alone by showing them that others are going through similar problems. Group therapy often takes one of three forms: **psychoeducational groups**, **therapy groups**, or **activity groups**.

> Group therapy allows patients to learn not only from the therapist, but also from the interactions between the therapist and other patients, and other patients and themselves. This form of psychosocial treatment also can help patients to feel less alone by showing them that others are going through similar problems.

Psychoeducational groups are helpful because they teach patients about their illness in a clear, structured way, similar to a small classroom. In psychoeducational groups, patients learn from mental health professionals about symptoms, treatments, early warning signs, and other topics relevant to psychosis.

Therapy groups focus more on helping patients explore their relationships, their coping styles, and stressors that may make symptoms worse. Rather than learning about symptoms and treatments, patients work on the parts of their own personality styles that may interfere with psychosocial success.

Activity groups are based on structured activities. Thus, the focus is less on learning or counseling and more on experiences and activities. These groups work on developing social skills, confidence, and in some cases, job-related skills.

Family Interventions

Families of patients in the early stages of psychosis often experience significant stress from the illness. Caregivers may lack social support while caring for an ill family member or may be concerned about the effects of the stigma associated with psychosis (see Chapter 12 on Fighting Stigma). Family interventions help families to cope with stress, improve their social supports, and reduce the effects of stigma. While we briefly review family interventions provided by mental health professionals here, Chapter 13 (Reducing Stress, Coping, and Communicating Effectively: Tips for Family Members and Patients) focuses on what patients and families can do to strengthen the family during this stressful time.

There are several forms of **family interventions**, all of which focus on helping the family as a whole rather than just the patient. Such interventions view each member of the family as having an important role or purpose. Without that member's involvement in the family system, the system would not work as well. Family interventions help both the patient and his or her family by involving each available member of the patient's immediate family. When one member of the family household becomes ill from a physical or mental illness, other family members experience some level of distress. In the same way, stress within the family often greatly affects the person with the illness. Family interventions can be divided into family psychoeducation and family therapy, though in many instances both of these occur in the same family intervention.

Family psychoeducation educates family members about early psychosis and the types of experiences that they can expect when a loved one has psychosis. Like individual psychoeducation or psychoeducational groups for patients themselves, family psychoeducation teaches family members about symptoms, diagnoses, evaluations, treatments, and other topics relevant to psychosis. Family psychoeducation may also focus on communication and problem-solving skills within the family. Additionally, and perhaps most importantly, family members learn to recognize the signs and symptoms of a relapse (early warning signs). They also learn strategies for reducing the chance of future relapses. Family psychoeducation may take place in several sessions over an extended period of time, sometimes with weekly or monthly meetings lasting 30–90 minutes. The series of sessions may last for several weeks or months.

Family psychoeducation is led by a mental health professional. It may take place within a single family. On the other hand, family psychoeducation may take place within **multi-family groups**, in which family members from several different families that are going through the same thing are present. Multi-family groups may be helpful because family members can talk to other families who also have a loved one experiencing a psychotic disorder. The patient may or may not be present when family psychoeducation takes place in multi-family groups.

Family therapy is another form of family intervention. Like family psychoeducation, family therapy may be helpful in reducing the chance of relapse or re-hospitalization after a first psychotic episode. This is because family therapy directly targets stressors in the patient's immediate environment. Research has shown that family stress may worsen the symptoms of someone in the early stages of psychosis, possibly leading to a relapse. Family therapy focuses not only on educating the family about psychosis (as in family psychoeducation), but also on improving communication and problem-solving skills. Family therapy strengthens the family's best coping skills, while minimizing problems and interaction styles that could create stress.

Supportive Housing

For some individuals with early psychosis, living alone or with family members is not feasible. This may be because the symptoms of psychosis interfere with their ability to maintain a household or because there are no family members available. In these cases, **supportive housing** options may be an alternative. Supportive housing provides people with serious mental illnesses a supportive and safe place to live. This could be a private apartment, an apartment shared with a roommate, or a group home. Staff members of supportive housing programs usually have knowledge of and experience with mental illnesses. However, such programs do not target symptoms directly. Instead, supportive housing focuses on assisting patients to become more independent in their living arrangements. Providing patients with this structure and support may help to decrease stress and move them towards a recovery path that includes independent living.

Supported Employment and Vocational Rehabilitation

Unfortunately, it is common for individuals with psychotic disorders to be unemployed and to have difficulty getting a job. In fact, around half of people with first-episode psychosis are unemployed. However, as a psychotic disorder progresses, this figure rises to more than 75% or three-fourths of people with psychosis. One way to help people with this problem is through a psychosocial treatment called **supported employment**. Supported employment is one type of the more general treatment approach called **vocational rehabilitation**. Vocational rehabilitation programs provide a variety of services, including vocational counseling and guidance, assessment of work skills and interests, training in particular job skills, support services (like transportation or interpreters), and assistance with job placement. So, these programs help individuals with psychosis find and keep jobs. Supported employment programs allow people with serious mental illnesses to work either part-time or full-time, while keeping job stress at a minimum. Supported employment programs try to place patients in the type of work that best fits them in terms of interest, skills, and comfort level. Just as supportive housing aims to move patients towards a recovery path that includes independent living, supported employment aims to move patients towards successful independent employment that provides them with an income.

Another approach that is being considered by some researchers is **supported education**. This would support patients with first-episode psychosis in late adolescence or early adulthood to complete their education. Most people who develop psychosis do so at an age that interrupts their schooling. Furthermore, in most societies the completion of high school is extremely important for future employment. So, education is an area of psychosocial functioning that often needs attention and support.

Social Skills Training

Social skills are the daily skills that allow us to successfully interact with one another and have rewarding relationships. As mentioned earlier, first-episode psychosis typically develops during late adolescence and early adulthood. During this time many young people are developing social skills and moving through key social milestones. For example, during this time, young people are graduating from high school, entering college, having their first romantic relationships, and getting their first jobs. Developing psychotic symptoms often disrupts the normal process of social development and interferes with these milestones. Patients with psychosis may have problems with social skills such as lacking assertiveness and finding it difficult to start a conversation.

Social skills training is a psychosocial treatment that helps patients to regain their prior level of social skills or to resume development of social skills interrupted by psychosis. Social skills training focuses on problem solving and works to increase social adjustment of patients with psychosis without necessarily focusing only on their symptoms. Like other psychosocial treatments, this form of treatment helps patients move towards recovery that is broader than just remission.

> Social skills training is a psychosocial treatment that helps patients to regain their prior level of social skills or to resume development of social skills interrupted by psychosis.

Social skills training is useful in teaching patients to communicate successfully, interact, and become more assertive. It teaches how to succeed in social interactions by breaking down complex social behaviors into smaller, easier-to-handle parts. This treatment can take place in many settings, including inpatient treatment groups, outpatient day programs, and individual therapy sessions. It may be given as a single group session, as an ongoing weekly treatment, or as a part of other psychosocial treatments like cognitive-behavioral therapy or group therapy. An important part of social skills training is repetition of the targeted skill. After learning the targeted skill, patients usually must practice it.

Assertive Community Treatment

Assertive community treatment (ACT) is a psychosocial treatment in which a team of mental health professionals brings treatment opportunities to patients in their own settings. For example, a psychiatrist, nurse, and social worker may visit the patient in his or her home rather than in a clinic setting. So, the basic premise of ACT programs is that the treatment team comes to the patient (at home), instead of the patient having to come to the treatment team (in a clinic). ACT teams help patients function at their best within their own community rather than in the hospital. These teams tend to have staff members who work with fewer patients than in other treatment settings. ACT is helpful in improving symptoms, reducing hospitalizations, and improving housing stability. There is typically no limit on the amount of time that a patient can receive ACT services. Unfortunately, ACT programs are not available in all communities, often because this treatment tends to be expensive for the health system.

Substance Abuse Treatment Programs

It is quite common for people experiencing a first episode of psychosis or another serious mental illness to have problems with substance abuse (see Chapter 10 on Staying Healthy). Substance abuse usually makes symptoms worse and recovery more difficult. Patients with psychosis who are dealing with a substance abuse problem have a **dual-diagnosis**, meaning that they have a diagnosis of both a psychotic disorder and a substance use disorder. Other terms sometimes used for dual-diagnosis are **comorbidity** or **co-occurring disorders**, which mean that two illnesses happen at the same time, in this case a psychotic disorder and an addiction. Dually diagnosed patients are more likely to have problems sticking with their medicine. They also have more social problems and have increased rates of relapse. As a result, the treatment of substance abuse, in addition to the treatment of psychosis, is critical.

As discussed in more detail in Chapter 10, mental health professionals may recommend specific programs that target substance abuse problems. Just two examples of such programs are 12-step programs and dual-diagnosis programs. Alcoholics Anonymous (AA) was the first **12-step program**. These types of programs now exist to help people with other problems including cigarette smoking and the use of illegal drugs. In 12-step programs, an individual follows an ordered list of increasingly challenging tasks that take them along the road towards recovery. In these programs, someone who has completed the 12 steps often guides a newcomer just beginning the steps through the program.

A **dual-diagnosis program** is a treatment program that focuses on individuals who not only have a diagnosed mental illness but also have a substance abuse problem. Such program are often in an inpatient or residential setting (meaning that the patient lives there for several weeks or months). These programs treat both problems. There are also outpatient dual-diagnosis programs in some communities. Such programs combine, or integrate, the treatment of psychosis with the treatment of substance abuse in the same program. For this reason, such programs are sometimes referred to as **integrated treatment programs**. This type of treatment reduces the possibility of conflicting messages or treatment goals from different treatment providers. Mental health professionals in these programs have a particular focus on the treatment of psychosis and substance abuse.

> A dual-diagnosis program is a treatment program that focuses on individuals who not only have a diagnosed mental illness but also have a substance abuse problem. Such programs are often in an inpatient or residential setting (meaning that the patient lives there for several weeks or months). These programs treat both problems.

Day Treatment Programs and Partial Hospitalization

Day treatment programs and **partial hospitalization** are outpatient treatment facilities that provide daytime (but not overnight) treatment to individuals diagnosed with psychosis and other mental illnesses. They often serve as a "step-down" program after an inpatient hospitalization. They also may provide a more intensive treatment than usual outpatient clinic appointments in order to prevent a hospitalization. These programs may be offered in combination with supportive housing and supported employment programs. Day treatment programs differ in the types of daily activities provided, but many of them offer a number of the psychosocial treatments discussed in this chapter. Both day treatment and partial hospitalization provide a fairly intensive form of treatment without requiring overnight hospital stays.

Putting It All Together

In addition to symptoms, patients may face other difficulties such as problems in work, school, relationships, or recreation and leisure activities. These psychosocial problems may occur when a person does not have the social skills necessary to successfully interact with his or her social environment. Psychosocial treatments aim to help patients to overcome psychosocial problems and resume psychosocial development that may have been delayed because of the time that psychotic symptoms usually appear, in late adolescence and early adulthood. Psychosocial treatments include cognitive-behavioral therapy, group therapy, family interventions, supportive housing, supported employment and vocational rehabilitation, social skills training, assertive community treatment, substance abuse treatment programs, and day treatment programs and partial hospitalization. Mental health professionals may recommend one of these treatments or combine several depending on the individual's needs.

Psychosocial treatments are most effective when patients have some insight into their illness and an adequate level of reality testing. However, sometimes having a good relationship with and trust in one's mental health professional is more important at the start of treatment. Families may be afraid to seek and begin treatment because they do not know what to expect. However, research shows that those who receive treatment early in psychosis respond better to treatment than those who have a longer period of untreated illness. This means that getting into effective treatment sooner may help to improve many problems associated with psychosis. Some have even argued that psychosocial treatments are more helpful during early psychosis than in later stages of illnesses like schizophrenia. This is because early intervention provides an opportunity to reduce symptoms before they become too severe, such as decreasing delusional ideas before they become a firmly held belief of the patient.

Worksheet 7.1 Psychosocial Treatments Included in the Treatment Plan

Here is a place to mark the psychosocial treatments that are included in the treatment plan. It is also a place to keep the names and contact information for each of those referrals.

Type of Treatment	Name of Program/ Center	Phone Number	Name of Person You Will Be Working With

Key Chapter Points

- ☛ Individuals experiencing a psychotic episode in late adolescence or early adulthood often experience an interruption in normal psychosocial development.
- ☛ The purpose of psychosocial treatments is to help patients change behaviors, by focusing on problems in interacting with their social environment.
- ☛ The time an individual with psychosis must stay in the various psychosocial treatments depends on the needs of that individual.
- ☛ Cognitive-behavioral therapy treats delusional ideas by helping the patient to consider alternative explanations and to learn behavioral experiments to test their belief system.
- ☛ Family interventions educate the family about psychosis, how to improve family communication, and problem-solving skills as a way of reducing stress in the family environment.
- ☛ Social skills training is useful in teaching patients to communicate, interact, and be more assertive.
- ☛ Dually diagnosed patients, with both psychosis and substance abuse, often have difficulty sticking with their medicine. They also have more social problems and have higher rates of relapse. So, substance abuse treatment is often very important.

Acknowledgments: This chapter was initially developed by Hanan D. Trotman, MA. Jean Addington, PhD, and Eóin Killackey, DPsych, served as collaborators for this chapter.

8

Follow-up and Sticking with Treatment

When someone is diagnosed with a first episode of psychosis, it can be easy to want to forget about the diagnosis after leaving the hospital or clinic. Symptoms may even appear to go away. However, the likely reason the person's symptoms have improved is that he or she has been taking medicine and getting treatment. It is important for the patient to stick to this treatment plan to continue to feel better, have decreasing symptoms, and eventually return to normal functioning.

Adherence

At the hospital or clinic, patients work with mental health professionals on a plan for their treatment. **Adherence** or **compliance** is when patients stick with their treatment plan and include this plan into their daily life. Mental health professionals use the words *adherence* and *compliance* to mean the same thing. In this book, we use the word adherence. Adherence includes: (1) attending follow-up appointments with mental health professionals, (2) taking medicine regularly, and (3) completing therapy exercises given at appointments (see Figure 8.1). We discuss each of these in the following pages.

Attending Follow-up Appointments

Before the patient leaves the hospital or clinic, the mental health professional and patient will discuss or plan future follow-up

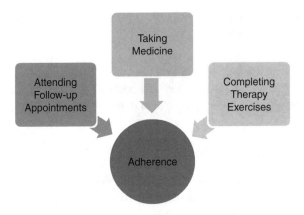

Figure 8.1 Adherence Includes Attending Follow-up Appointments, Taking Medicine, and Completing Therapy Exercises Given at Appointments

appointments. Patients may need to go to these appointments every other week, or even more frequently, when just leaving the hospital. Those who have stayed well for a longer period may be able to go to appointments less often. They may go every month and eventually, only every three months. If available in the community, other choices may include appointments in the home or in the community with case managers or treating professionals (See Chapter 7 on Psychosocial Treatments for Early Psychosis).

Appointments may be at a clinic or hospital and usually last 30 to 45 minutes. They may be with a doctor for a checkup. The patient also may have to go to appointments for counseling, therapy, or other types of psychosocial treatments. The number of appointments the patient has to go to will depend on his or her specific needs. Knowing that they have to go to many sessions may be disappointing for patients. Most people do not like going to the doctor! This is true for many people with psychosis as well.

Not wanting to go to see a mental health professional for ongoing follow-up is understandable. However, these appointments are very helpful in many ways. For example, they allow an experienced mental health professional to monitor the patient's illness. They also allow the patient and the mental health professional to continue building a strong working relationship. And they provide a supportive environment in which patients can talk about their concerns, stresses, and goals for recovery.

> Not wanting to go to see a mental health professional for ongoing follow-up is understandable. However, these appointments are very helpful in many ways.

Taking Medicine Regularly

Medicine adherence is very important to help treat psychotic symptoms. Research has proven that antipsychotics can help to relieve and reduce psychotic symptoms, sometimes completely or to a point that they do not affect daily activities. In addition to treating symptoms, medicines are also important in preventing another episode of psychosis. So, it is necessary to continue taking the medicine even when things are going well and the symptoms have gone away.

However, like other medicines, antipsychotics may have unpleasant side effects. It is important to understand that medicine is a very necessary part of the treatment plan. Patients may need reminders to take their medicine because of psychotic symptoms they may be experiencing. They may not see the reason to keep taking their medicine once symptoms are reduced or relieved. Sometimes, they do not realize that they need medicine to keep them well or that they even have a mental health problem (see Chapter 2 on What Are the Symptoms of Psychosis?).

As noted above regarding follow-up appointments, it is understandable that many patients do not like to take medicine. Most people would not like having to take a pill every day. It can be a hassle, and it is a daily reminder that one has an illness. However, taking the medicine clearly helps to reduce symptoms. It also makes recovery and pursuing one's life goals easier given that symptoms will be under control. Furthermore, continuing the medicine reduces the chance of having a relapse and possibly having to go to the hospital again. For more information on medicine, see Chapter 6 on Medicines Used to Treat Psychosis.

Completing Therapy Exercises

Sometimes mental health professionals use certain forms of therapy in addition to medicines. Some of these forms of therapy, like cognitive-behavioral therapy, give "homework assignments." These therapy exercises help the patient to understand the symptoms they are experiencing. They also help the patient develop coping skills to deal with the symptoms and with stress. Because of this, it is important to adhere to the treatment plan and complete these recommended exercises.

Mental Health Treatment Plans

Adherence with the treatment plan for the first episode of psychosis is the same as with any other medical treatment plan. For example, if you have diabetes you must attend follow-up appointments regularly so that the doctor can monitor your symptoms and blood sugar levels. Someone with hypertension (high blood pressure) has to take medicine regularly in order to keep the blood pressure low and prevent it from becoming too high again. If you have a broken leg, you have to complete physical therapy exercises in order to strengthen your leg so that you can walk and run again without pain. In the case of early psychosis, adherence includes: (1) attending follow-up appointments with mental health professionals, (2) taking medicine regularly, and (3) completing therapy exercises given at appointments. One of the long-term goals of treatment is to help individuals take care of their own illness just like people with diabetes must learn to do.

Time in Treatment

When you break a leg, they put on a cast for a certain amount of time. After they remove the cast, the doctors recommend an exercise plan and follow-up appointments. You might also see a physical therapist to help the healing process. The necessary follow-up for a broken leg takes less time than for many medical illnesses. For example, diabetes and hypertension are often lifelong illnesses. They require follow-up for a longer period. If you have diabetes, you may have to change your lifestyle and daily schedule in order to stay healthy. You must follow a strict diet, regularly take your medicine, and check your blood sugar level. You also will have to attend regular appointments so that the doctor can monitor your health.

Just as physical health issues require different lengths of time for follow-up, so do mental health issues. Sometimes people diagnosed with a first episode of psychosis will have to be in treatment for a shorter period, such as when you break a leg. However, most people who experience a first episode of psychosis will have to continue for longer, like those with diabetes.

> Sometimes people diagnosed with a first episode of psychosis will have to be in treatment for a shorter period, such as when you break a leg. However, most people who experience a first episode of psychosis will have to continue for longer, like those with diabetes.

Nonadherence

Sometimes patients are **nonadherent**. This means they do not stick with their treatment plan or make this plan part of their daily life. They may not attend their follow-up appointments. They also may not take their medicine regularly or complete their therapy exercises.

Patients may be nonadherent for many reasons. Some reasons are:

- They may simply forget to take their medicine.
- They may not want a reminder of their illness by having to take medicines every day or by even talking about their illness.
- They may not believe that they have a mental health problem.
- They may distrust those around them because of certain symptoms, like paranoia, which may make them less willing to follow their treatment plan.
- They may not be able to afford their medicine and/or follow-up services.
- They may not want to deal with the side effects of the medicine.
- They may not want to take the time to attend appointments.
- They may have transportation problems that make it hard to attend follow-up appointments.
- They may lack support from others such as family and friends.

- They may be using substances regularly, which interferes with their ability to stick to their treatment plan.

Importance of Adherence

Research has shown that nonadherence makes it about five times more likely that patients will relapse with similar or more severe symptoms. Relapse could lead to a stay in a hospital, and it usually takes a longer time to respond to treatment each time there is a relapse. Adherence with the treatment plan is important because it decreases the chances of relapse and is the best way to prevent hospitalization (see Figure 8.2). However, even people who adhere to their treatment plan sometimes have a relapse of psychotic symptoms. Such a relapse may be related to substance abuse such as using marijuana (see Chapter 10 on Staying Healthy). It may be due to stressful life events. For some people, it may be the natural course of the illness.

> Adherence with the treatment plan is important because it decreases the chances of relapse and is the best way to prevent hospitalization.

Hospitalization

Some people may decide to go to a hospital for treatment if they start to have symptoms again. In such cases, if they are hospitalized, it is called voluntary hospitalization. Others may need involuntary

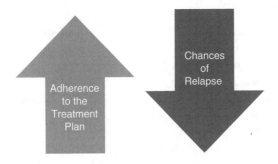

Figure 8.2 Adherence to Treatment Decreases the Chances of Relapse

hospitalization if their symptoms cause them to be a threat to themselves or others or if their symptoms become severe. Involuntary hospitalization may be of use when the patient's safety or another's safety is at risk. Again, adherence is the best way to shorten time in the hospital or avoid another stay. Whether in the hospital, just coming out of the hospital, or in treatment in an outpatient clinic setting, the support of family and friends can do a lot to help people who have experienced a first episode of psychosis to stick to their treatment plan.

Support from Family and Friends

Family and friends can help improve adherence. Support from others can help patients remember their appointments and medicine. They can also help encourage patients because they want what is best for them. Sometimes people who are experiencing psychosis have impaired insight and may not fully understand their diagnosis. They may not understand what would help them to feel and function better. Family members are able to recognize the need for follow-up appointments when patients sometimes cannot.

Family and friends should try to understand the patient's treatment plan so that they can help the patient with adherence. The worksheet at the end of Chapter 6 helps to keep track of the patient's medicines and the worksheet at the end of Chapter 7 helps keep track of psychosocial treatments.

Tips for Family and Friends

There are many ways that family and friends can encourage adherence. A few examples are:

- Make a plan with the patient for ways to help, especially if he or she becomes nonadherent.
- Listen to the patient and try to be understanding of his or her issues or concerns.
- Help the patient with medicine adherence by counting the pills in their bottles, if need be. However, it is important not to appear too controlling.
- Watch the patient take the medicine or ask if he or she took it, if need be.
- Use helpful reminders such as a daily or weekly pill container.

- Attend follow-up appointments with the patient.

Usually, it is best not to try to force or trick patients into taking their medicine. This could make some symptoms, like distrust or paranoia, worse.

Support for Family and Friends

Family and friends who are supporting someone with a first episode of psychosis need support themselves. This is a difficult time, and it helps to connect with others who understand how difficult and frightening dealing with this illness can be. Mental health professionals can help family and friends to connect with others who have dealt with these same issues. These connections can be with individuals or with organizations such as the National Alliance on Mental Illness (NAMI) and Mental Health America (MHA) in the United States. Other countries have similar organizations to provide support for families and friends. These persons or organizations can provide information as well as support.

Putting It All Together

Sticking to one's treatment plan is important to continue to feel better, have less symptoms, and eventually return to normal functioning. The three parts of adherence are attending follow-up appointments with mental health professionals, taking medicine regularly, and completing therapy exercises given at appointments. While the time in treatment will differ for different individuals, most people with psychosis will have to continue treatment for a long period of time. There are many reasons patients may be nonadherent, such as an unwillingness to accept their illness, the symptoms themselves, impaired insight, and time and costs of treatment. Even though adherence will be difficult at times for these and other reasons, adherence decreases the chances of relapse and rehospitalization. Support both from and for family and friends is important in helping patients to stick with treatment (see Chapter 13 on Reducing Stress, Coping, and Communicating Effectively: Tips for Family Members and Patients). The next chapter discusses how to recognize the early warning signs of a relapse and work to avoid rehospitalization (see Chapter 9)

Key Chapter Points

- ☞ Adherence is when patients stick with their treatment plan and make this plan part of their daily life.
- ☞ Adherence includes attending follow-up appointments, taking medicine, and completing therapy exercises given at appointments.
- ☞ Even though having to go to a clinic or hospital for many sessions may be disappointing for patients, these appointments are meant to help them stay well.
- ☞ Medicine adherence is very important to help treat psychotic symptoms and help patients avoid hospitalization.
- ☞ Sometimes people diagnosed with a first episode of psychosis will have to be in treatment for a short period; others will have to continue longer.
- ☞ Research has shown that nonadherence increases the chances that patients will relapse with similar or more severe symptoms than before.
- ☞ Family and friends should try to understand the patient's treatment plan so that they can help the patient with adherence.
- ☞ Adherence is the best way to shorten time in the hospital or avoid hospitalization altogether.

Acknowledgments: This chapter was initially developed by Erin M. Bergner, MPH. Ashok Malla, MBBS, FRCPC, MRCPsych, and Srividya N. Iyer, PhD, served as collaborators for this chapter.

III   Helping You Look Ahead to Next Steps

9

Early Warning Signs and Preventing a Relapse

In this chapter, we discuss **early warning signs**, which are signs and symptoms that often occur before an episode of psychosis. These signs and symptoms, though mild, may occur before the first episode of psychosis and also before later episodes. That is, some mild signs and symptoms may occur during the prodromal phase of the illness, before psychotic symptoms first develop. These same signs and symptoms often serve as warning signs before another episode of illness, or a **relapse** of psychosis, occurs. So, it is important to be familiar with early warning signs and what to do if they begin to develop.

The Importance of Detecting Early Warning Signs

Many people who have had a first episode of psychosis will go on to have one or more relapses of their illness. A relapse happens when symptoms appear again. Some relapses may happen with little or no warning over a short period of time, such as a few days. However, most relapses develop slowly over longer periods, like a few weeks. A relapse may or may not require hospitalization, but it definitely calls for immediate attention, evaluation, and treatment. After a stay in the hospital or after outpatient stabilization, some people feel better quickly. Others take weeks, or even months, to function as well as they had before the relapse.

One way of avoiding a relapse is to stay in treatment and attend all follow-up appointments (see Chapter 8 on Follow-up and Sticking with Treatment). Also, it is very important to become aware of one's specific early warning signs, which are changes in thoughts, feelings, and behaviors that happen a few days or weeks before an episode (reappearance of symptoms). By carefully watching for these signs, patients, their families, and their mental health professionals can work together to help lessen the severity of any episode that may occur. **Relapse prevention** is the goal of preventing a relapse altogether, by sticking to treatment and watching for early warning signs.

The first step in determining one's specific early warning signs is to think back to the changes that occurred in the prodromal period of the illness, or the time just before the *first* episode of psychosis. While there are common early warning signs, they will show up slightly differently in each person. Early warning signs in one person may be clear and easy to detect, while in another person they may be trickier to figure out. Early warning signs are signals that symptoms are beginning again and that another episode of psychosis may happen.

> Early warning signs in one person may be clear and easy to detect, while in another person they may be trickier to figure out. Early warning signs are signals that symptoms are beginning again and that another episode of psychosis may happen.

Common Early Warning Signs

Even though each person experiences symptoms that may be somewhat unique, there are some common early warning signs experienced by many people with psychosis. For some people, some of the common early warning signs (like social withdrawal, avolition, and decreased expression of emotion, each of which is described below) continue after a psychotic episode has resolved. As such, they may be long-lasting and not necessarily a warning sign for another psychotic episode. Common early warning signs include:

- *Mood Changes—Sadness, Tension, or Irritability:* Sadness, also called **dysphoria**, may be an early warning sign for some people who have had an episode of psychosis. They may express this sadness as feeling "blue," "down," sad, discouraged, hopeless, distressed, or uninterested in their usual pastimes. Tension may look like anxiety, nervousness, worry, or restlessness (such as an inability to sit still or pacing back and forth). Some people may also come across as hostile, angry, or irritable (feeling touchy, impatient, or on edge).

- *Sleep Disturbance:* People with a sleep disturbance may have insomnia, hypersomnia, or even day/night reversal. **Insomnia** is a difficulty in falling asleep or staying asleep. For example, insomnia may be defined as taking more than 30 minutes to fall asleep or waking up in the middle of the night and not being able to go back to sleep. It can also be waking up more than 30 minutes earlier than wanted in the morning. The opposite of this is **hypersomnia**, when the person sleeps more than usual. Unlike insomnia and hypersomnia, people with **day/night reversal** get about the same amount of sleep as usual but stay awake at night and sleep during the day.

- *Ideas of Reference:* Ideas of reference occur when people think that others are talking about them or referring to them when they really are not. For example, a person may think that someone on the radio or the television is speaking about or trying to send coded messages to him or her. Unlike in a delusion (see Chapter 2 on What Are the Symptoms of Psychosis?), he or she may partly recognize that these beliefs could be wrong.

- *Suspiciousness:* People who are suspicious feel that others cannot be trusted. They may have an unexplained feeling that those around them are trying to cause problems in their life. For example, they may think that other people are plotting against them or cheating, harassing, or even trying to harm them in some way. However, unlike paranoia, they may partly recognize that their beliefs may be wrong. Even still, people with suspiciousness may begin to isolate themselves from others because they do not feel that they can trust people. An example of suspiciousness is thinking that strangers at a shopping mall are laughing at and talking about you or that someone is out to get you for no reason at all. It is important to remember that this is only an early warning sign if it is different from how the person normally behaves or thinks. Experiencing suspiciousness may be an early warning sign that more serious paranoia is about to develop.

- *Unusual Ideas:* For people to have unusual ideas as an early warning sign, the ideas must be a change from the way they normally think. People may be confused over what is real or imaginary, have **overvalued ideas**, or have **magical thinking**. Unlike a full delusion, people may realize that their ideas are either untrue or are an exaggeration of what is really going on. An overvalued idea is when too much emphasis is placed on an idea. Overvalued ideas can involve religious or philosophical thoughts or may involve some other idea that one is overly concerned with. Magical thinking can involve such things as wondering about the ability to read others' minds or believing too much in superstitions.

- ***Trouble Thinking or Concentrating:*** People experiencing this sign have problems with their thought process, or the way their thoughts work. They may become less able to organize their thoughts and speech. That is, because they are having trouble with their thinking, they may have trouble with speaking and making themselves clear. They also may become less able to concentrate, to focus their attention, or to communicate with others. At times, they may have difficulty understanding what others are saying to them. They also may experience thought blocking, or an interruption in the flow of thought. In other words, they seem to get "off track" or cannot put their thoughts into words. As a result, they may be very slow to respond to questions or may not respond at all.

- ***Perceptual Abnormalities:*** A **perceptual abnormality** is when the experience of one of the five senses (hearing, seeing, feeling, tasting, or smelling) changes enough that the person wonders if the mind might be playing tricks on him or her. Examples include mistaking the rustling of leaves for voices talking, hearing one's name called in a noisy room, briefly seeing someone else's face when looking in a mirror, seeing something out of the corner of one's eye incorrectly, or thinking that spots on the wall at first glance look like bugs.

- ***Brief, Intermittent Hallucinations:*** A hallucination is a more serious form of perceptual abnormality, occurring when one senses something that does not actually exist. Examples of **brief, intermittent hallucinations** include hearing a name called out loud that no one else can hear or seeing an object or person for a few seconds that no one else can see. Unlike a full hallucination that can happen once psychosis has developed, a brief, intermittent hallucination happens only occasionally and lasts only a few seconds to several minutes. Brief, intermittent hallucinations may be an early warning sign that hallucinations are about to develop again.

- *Deterioration in Role Functioning:* A **deterioration in role functioning** is said to occur when people become less able to carry out daily activities. These activities can include work, family responsibilities, household chores, personal hygiene, recreation, and socializing. For example, there could be a drop in grades or less social interaction. Others may begin to notice an unusually strong body odor due to poor hygiene. An employer may criticize or fire a person who no longer seems to be working as hard as he or she used to. These are all forms of deterioration in role functioning, which in some cases may be an early warning sign for another psychotic episode in someone who has had a first episode of psychosis.

- *Social Withdrawal:* People who have **social withdrawal** are generally not interested in having social contact with others and are less likely to become involved socially. It can appear as if they are pulling back from social situations or that they have poor social skills. Even if they will still join in on social activities when others approach them, they will hardly ever seek out socializing opportunities themselves. This may happen because they feel less comfortable around others or because they are developing positive or negative symptoms.

- *Avolition:* **Avolition** is a significant decrease in the motivation or ability to begin and/or follow through with tasks. People with avolition may be unable to finish tasks or complete them on time. When avolition is severe, it keeps people from completing many different types of tasks. As a result, they may neglect work, school, and/or family responsibilities. In addition, people may also stop taking care of their personal hygiene such as bathing, combing their hair, and changing their clothes. Like social withdrawal, avolition may be a negative symptom that precedes another psychotic episode.

- *Decreased Expression of Emotion:* It is important to keep in mind that normal expression of emotions differs from person to person. Normally, people express emotions through facial expressions, gestures, body language, and the pitch, tone, and rate of speech. **Decreased expression of emotion**, which is also called blunted affect, happens when there is a change or lessening in their "usual" expression of emotion. While a decreased expression of emotion may be obvious to others, many people experiencing this sign are unaware of how they are presenting themselves.

- **Other Early Warning Signs:** There may be other significant changes in thought, behavior, or emotion that signal that a relapse of psychosis is about to happen. In general, these are things that seem "out of character" for the person. Examples of other early warning signs include not answering the phone, eating too little or too much, or making a sudden, drastic change in one's appearance.

Relapse Prevention: Responding to Early Warning Signs

It is quite common to experience one or more early warning signs just before an episode of psychosis. While there are common early warning signs, some may be unique to each person. It is important to keep in mind that each person with psychosis will not experience all of the early warning signs discussed earlier. People who have experienced an episode of psychosis should try to remember the two or three early warning signs that may be their unique signals that problems may be recurring. One person's early warning signs may be insomnia, irritability, and being argumentative. Another person's may be perceptual abnormalities and brief, intermittent hallucinations. Yet another person's early warning signs may be suspiciousness and social withdrawal. It is helpful for mental health professionals, family, and the individual's other supports to be aware of the individual's particular early warning signs.

By carefully observing changes, people have a better chance of responding quickly enough to these early warning signs so that patients spend less time in the hospital—or even avoid hospitalization. Recognizing and reacting quickly to these signs is the main goal of monitoring them. There are a few important steps to take when responding to early warning signs, as discussed below and shown in Figure 9.1.

> By carefully observing changes, people have a better chance of responding quickly enough to these early warning signs so that patients spend less time in the hospital—or even avoid hospitalization.

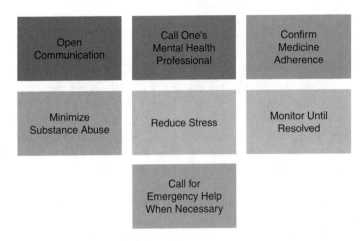

Figure 9.1 Steps to Take when Reposonding to Early Warning Signs

- *Open Communication.* If it seems that early warning signs are developing, it is critical for that person and his or her family or supports to meet to openly discuss these concerns. During that discussion, other explanations for the changes can be considered. The main goal of discussing these issues is to figure out if these changes may actually be early warning signs of a relapse. If so, it is important to begin extra measures to reduce the chance of a relapse.

- *Call One's Mental Health Professional.* The individual and his or her family should meet with the mental health professional. The psychiatrist will want to meet to decide if it is necessary to temporarily increase the dose of medicine. To determine if the dosage is adequate, the doctor may need to draw blood to check medicine levels. The doctor will also want to assess for side effects. At times, the patient will need to switch to a different medicine. The treatment team also may recommend adding or increasing a psychosocial treatment (see Chapter 7). If it seems that a relapse is coming, it is important to not wait until the next regularly scheduled appointment. After noticing early warning signs, prescribing additional medicine within a few days is an important step for preventing a relapse and hospitalization.

- **Confirm Medicine Adherence.** Early warning signs and relapse often happen after a person has decreased his or her medicine or stopped taking medicine altogether. It is important to check the patient's medicine plan as soon as early warning signs appear. Family and friends can ask the person directly or can count his or her pills. If the person has not taken his or her medicine properly, it is time to increase monitoring, reminders, and encouragement for taking medicine as prescribed. At this time, it is also important to ask if the person feels that they are having any side effects that may be caused by taking the medicines, and if so, to look for a solution to these.

- **Minimize Substance Abuse.** Substance abuse can increase a person's risk of relapse. It is important to find out if substance abuse is a problem by asking the person directly and by observing the person. With alcohol abuse, he or she may smell of alcohol at times, have poor balance or slurred speech at times, and may begin to have problems functioning. In the case of street drugs, the smell of marijuana may be present. Finding paraphernalia such as rolling papers, cut plastic tubes, empty vials, and small plastic baggies may be a clue about drug use. Efforts should be made to minimize substance abuse. It is important to contact mental health providers for their advice and help with dealing with substance abuse. It may be necessary to have an evaluation by a substance abuse counselor as well (see Chapter 10 on Staying Healthy).

- **Reduce Stress.** A person who is at risk for experiencing another episode of psychosis is often very sensitive to stressful situations, such as arguments, criticism, and sudden increases in responsibility. Unfortunately, it can be difficult to evaluate stress levels because many people are not fully aware that they are under stress. They may even deny that it is a problem. It is also important to remember that stress does not cause all relapses. In addition, what is stressful for one person is not necessarily stressful for another. A person can respond to stress by reducing the source of the stress itself or by coping better with the stress that exists. Reducing stress can be achieved by cutting back on responsibilities, looking for new enjoyable and relaxing activities to participate in, or dealing with a conflict or problem that is causing worry. Coping with stress can involve relaxation techniques, talking with a counselor, participating in recreational activities, or becoming a part of a support group.

- ***Monitor Until Resolved.*** Once the patient and others recognize the problems and take steps to address these, it is important to monitor or watch early warning signs until there is obvious improvement. It is also important to continue meeting frequently with one's mental health professional to discuss progress. These meetings will provide important information about whether or not the patient has avoided a relapse. They also can provide information to reflect back on, if in the future there are other similar changes of behavior that are of concern. While monitoring, it is important to avoid making a person feel spied on or as if other people are "walking on eggshells" around him or her since this can be stressful. Family members should try to keep routines as normal as possible.

- ***Call for Emergency Help When Necessary.*** Sometimes, it may be necessary to call for emergency help if psychosis develops and the person exhibits behaviors that may be dangerous. For example, if the person threatens to harm him- or herself, or actually does something to harm him- or herself or others, it may be necessary to call for a mobile crisis unit, an ambulance, or at times, even police assistance. If the person is unable to care for his or her own health or safety, emergency help may be necessary. Sometimes, when psychosis develops and insight is impaired, it may be necessary for the person to go into the hospital. Most state/provincial or national governments have laws that allow doctors or the courts to hospitalize individuals against their will (involuntary hospitalization) if it is necessary to protect the individual and/or others. When it is necessary, hospitalization allows for more intensive short-term treatment of psychosis in a secure setting.

Putting It All Together

Even though many people who have experienced psychosis have relapses, it is possible to reduce the severity of relapses and even to prevent them. Therefore, after symptoms of the first episode of psychosis go away (remission), it is important to shift the focus to not just treatment, but also relapse prevention and recovery (see Chapter 11). Becoming aware of the early warning signs that are specific to a person who has had an episode of psychosis can help in monitoring for the possibility of a relapse. Monitoring helps the treatment team, family, and others to assist with reducing the problems that he or she is experiencing. By being familiar with and acting on early warning signs, a person may have less severe symptoms if a relapse does occur or may completely avoid a relapse. When responding to early warning signs it is important to communicate openly, call one's mental health professional, confirm medicine adherence, minimize substance abuse, reduce stress, monitor until resolved, and call for emergency help when necessary.

The following worksheet will help you to record and keep track of the early warning signs experienced in the past or present. It is also a place for you to keep comments and questions to discuss with your mental health professional.

Worksheet 9.1 Common Early Warning Signs

Common Early Warning Signs Place a check next to signs experienced.	✓	Questions or Comments Make note of any questions or comments you may have for your mental health professional.
Sadness		
Tension		
Irritability		
Sleep Disturbance		
Ideas of Reference		
Suspiciousness		
Unusual Ideas		
Trouble Thinking or Concentrating		
Perceptual Abnormalities		
Brief, Intermittent Hallucinations		
Deterioration in Role Functioning		
Social Withdrawal		
Avolition		
Decreased Expression of Emotion		
Other:		

Key Chapter Points

- ☞ A relapse happens when symptoms get much worse or when old symptoms appear again.
- ☞ Many people have one or more relapses of their illness.
- ☞ By carefully monitoring early warning signs, patients, their families, and their mental health professionals can work together to help lessen the severity of any episode that a person may have—or prevent a relapse altogether.

Acknowledgments: This chapter was initially developed by Sandra M. Goulding, MPH. Kristin Cadenhead, MD, served as a collaborator for this chapter.

10 Staying Healthy

To move towards recovery after a first episode of psychosis, patients must focus on both their mental and physical health. People with a serious mental illness are usually less healthy than those without such an illness. This may be because of the illness itself, fewer opportunities for health care, or unwanted effects of the medicines taken to treat mental illnesses. People with a long-lasting mental illness sometimes also deal with other issues, such as cigarette smoking, drug abuse, unhealthy eating habits, little exercise, and having few relationships with others. Even though it can be difficult at times, living a healthy lifestyle is necessary for patients to feel better and move towards recovery. In this chapter, we discuss problems sometimes faced by people with psychosis and ways to deal with and overcome these issues. Specifically, this chapter focuses on the importance of not smoking cigarettes, staying away from alcohol and drugs, having a healthy diet, getting plenty of exercise, and having good social support from family and friends.

Cigarette Smoking

One problem sometimes faced by people with psychosis is cigarette smoking. About one in five people in the general population in the United States (about 21%) smoke cigarettes. Fortunately, this percentage is now decreasing because of the growing awareness of the health risks posed by cigarette smoking. However, a large percentage of people with psychosis smoke. For example, most people with schizophrenia (between 50% and 90%) smoke cigarettes (see Figure 10.1). What's more, this percentage has not decreased in recent years.

People with psychotic disorders also have smoking behaviors that can cause even greater harm. Some of these behaviors include smoking heavily—up to two or three packs a day—and smoking cigarettes down to the filter where the greatest concentration of nicotine is.

Why are people with psychosis so likely to smoke, and to smoke so heavily? Most researchers believe that it is because of the relationship between cigarette smoking, nicotine, and the symptoms of psychosis (see Chapter 2 on What Are the Symptoms of Psychosis?). Nicotine is a drug that affects anyone who uses it. In most people, nicotine may slightly improve attention and memory. However, nicotine may have additional effects in people with psychosis. In addition to improving attention and memory, it also may subtly affect the symptoms of psychosis. Some research has shown that people with psychosis who smoke cigarettes actually have more severe positive and negative symptoms. So, they may be smoking to try to reduce these symptoms. Patients sometimes describe an increase in attention and motivation and

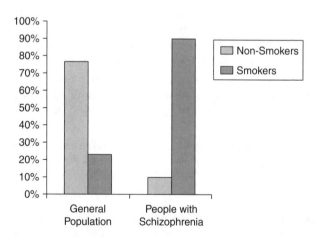

Figure 10.1 Percentage of People in the General Population Who Smoke Cigarettes Compared to the Percentage of People with Schizophrenia Who Smoke Cigarettes

a decrease in anxiety and tension when they smoke cigarettes. People with psychosis who are socially withdrawn or might not interact with others may find it easier to make friends while smoking cigarettes, especially in community centers or group homes. There are probably other complex reasons why people with psychosis are so likely to smoke.

Cigarette smoking causes the same harm to people with psychosis as it does to anyone else. People who smoke are at higher risk for smoking-related illnesses, such as emphysema, chronic bronchitis, heart disease, and lung cancer. Because more people with psychosis smoke, these illnesses affect people with psychosis more than they affect the general population.

In addition, cigarette smoking may interfere with the way the body processes some antipsychotic medicines used to treat psychosis (see Chapter 6 on Medicines Used to Treat Psychosis). Smoking can speed up the metabolism or breakdown of some of these medicines. In other words, smoking causes some of these medicines to pass through the body more quickly. Because of this, people with psychosis who smoke may require higher doses of certain medicines to treat their symptoms. The chances of side effects from these medicines increase with higher doses. If more side effects are experienced, a person might be less likely to adhere to his or her medicine (see Chapter 8 on Follow-up and Sticking with Treatment). For these reasons, along with the more obvious health risks, it is important for people with psychosis to quit or reduce their smoking.

Smoking cessation is the process of quitting smoking. **Nicotine replacement therapy** can be very helpful for someone trying to stop smoking. Smoking cessation programs typically offer nicotine replacement in the form of a gum, patch, or inhaler. These non-dangerous substitutions make it easier to quit smoking. Another treatment to help patients quit smoking is **motivational enhancement therapy**, which aims to increase one's desire or motivation to quit. Additionally, several **smoking cessation medicines**, including bupropion (Wellbutrin, Zyban) and varenicline (Chantix), are now available to make quitting easier. All of these treatments (nicotine replacement, motivational enhancement techniques, and smoking cessation medicines) work well together to help a person successfully quit smoking.

It is very important for young people who are experiencing a first episode of psychosis who smoke to seriously consider quitting smoking. Paying attention to mental and physical health early in psychosis can help patients to learn how to manage their illness without using substances. There are many places to turn to for help to quit smoking, but this process should be discussed with the patient's clinicians. To find helpful programs, one of the first places to check is the hospital or outpatient center where the patient receives mental health treatment. Often, the mental health professional (see Chapter 5 on The Initial Evaluation of Psychosis) can refer the patient to a local program. Family and friends are an important source of support.

> Paying attention to mental and physical health early in psychosis can help patients to learn how to manage their illness without using substances.

Substance Abuse

As with cigarette smoking, more people with psychosis abuse alcohol and other drugs than the general population. Around half (50%) of people with schizophrenia have a **substance use disorder**, or an addiction. A much lower percentage of the general population (about 17%) has an addiction (see Figure 10.2). People receive a diagnosis of a substance use disorder when the use of a substance interferes with their ability to perform on the job, disrupts healthy relationships, or results in legal problems. Abused substances can include alcohol or other drugs like marijuana, cocaine, methamphetamine, ecstasy, heroin, ketamine, PCP, and LSD.

There are several reasons why people with psychosis are more likely to abuse substances. Many mental health professionals believe that these individuals use alcohol and drugs to be more social, enhance their pleasure, cope with their symptoms, or try to self-medicate. This is very similar to the reasons why people with psychosis smoke cigarettes.

Many people use substances when in social situations. Because people with psychosis are often withdrawn (perhaps due to negative symptoms), using substances provides them with an opportunity to socialize with others. In addition, substance use enhances their pleasure because of the "high" that comes from using. This might be

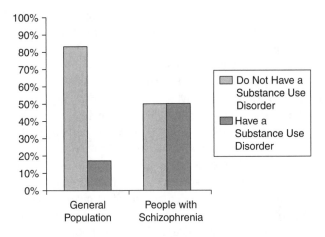

Figure 10.2 Percentage of People in the General Population Who Have a Diagnosis of a Substance Use Disorder Compared to the Percentage of People with Schizophrenia Who Have a Diagnosis of a Substance Use Disorder

a positive experience for people with psychosis because they may have diminished emotions, few close relationships, and minimal participation in social activities. Finally, people with psychosis use substances to cope with or try to self-medicate their symptoms. Substances sometimes relieve feelings of sadness and anxiety or help the patient to deal with severe symptoms like hallucinations or delusions. However, in the end, using drugs often actually makes these symptoms worse.

Even though using substances can be enjoyable for someone with psychosis, there are many negative and harmful effects on the body and the brain. Many drugs are both physically and mentally addictive. This means that drugs can affect the body, and coming off drugs can cause physical symptoms (like shaking, sweating, or high blood pressure). They can also affect the mind, and coming off drugs can cause psychological symptoms (like anxiety, insomnia, and irritability). As mentioned earlier, drugs also often make symptoms worse instead of better. Chronic alcohol use can lead to depression and liver damage and can negatively affect the metabolism of medicines, or the way they are absorbed into and work in the body. Most addictive drugs can make the symptoms of psychosis worse and interfere with its treatments. People who have experienced a first episode of psychosis are at higher risk for relapse or having another episode of psychosis if they use drugs. This may be especially true of certain drugs, like cocaine and methamphetamine.

It is important to try to prevent substance use in people with psychosis because they are at greater risk for abusing alcohol and drugs. Many people with psychosis who abuse substances begin long before the onset or start of their illness, which may play a role in the development of psychosis in some cases. However, others begin using substances after their illness has developed to try to cope with the symptoms. Patients benefit from having someone to regularly monitor their symptoms and from frequently speaking with their doctor about how they are feeling. Often, doctors can adjust medicines in order to help the patient feel better, and, hopefully, the patient will then not find it is necessary to turn to addictive substances. Doctors also can provide the best information about how substances affect someone's illness.

Family and friends may need to help monitor symptoms. It is helpful for patients if family and friends support them through their struggle. Providing a healthy, loving relationship can help them avoid drugs and alcohol entirely. In addition, participating in healthy activities with friends can help prevent the start of substance use and abuse.

Although prevention is preferred, even those who have already begun to use and abuse substances can quit. It will be difficult and it may take time. However, in the end, quitting will improve their mind, body, and illness. Patients should talk with their doctor about quitting. The doctor or other mental health professional can send them to the right therapist or program to help begin and maintain this necessary change. Their mental health professional also can help them stop using substances safely, because quitting some substances, like alcohol or heroin, suddenly can be dangerous or physically painful. However, quitting can be accomplished and should be an important priority. In some cases, a referral to a drug abuse specialist, like an addiction counselor, may be necessary. A specialist may do an evaluation and make recommendations on how to best treat the substance abuse problem. Such treatments may range from attending meetings (like Alcoholics Anonymous or Narcotics Anonymous), an intensive outpatient program, or even a long-term residential program, where people live in a structured recovery setting for six months or more.

Some of the steps to helping someone overcome substance abuse include: (1) understanding the change process, (2) keeping communication open, and (3) providing support at every possible opportunity. Understanding the change process is one of the most important steps to begin helping someone quit. Individuals often have to go through stages of change to quit. These stages include becoming aware of the problem, thinking about the change, beginning the change, and then maintaining that change long-term (see Figure 10.3). It is important to understand that this is a gradual process. Pushing someone to quit too quickly or being too hard on him or her will not help to stop the drug abuse. It is important for family and friends to remain supportive of the person through this process and not push him or her away. However, as described in Chapter 13, family members must also maintain their own health and reduce their own stress. Some families feel that there is a point at which they can no longer tolerate some behaviors like drug use. This sometimes means that families find it necessary to take measures to get the patient into substance abuse treatment.

Keeping communication open is also very important. The patient has to feel comfortable and free to talk about the difficulties of quitting. This open communication provides much needed support. It also allows family and friends a chance to express their concerns about the patient's well-being and future. For someone who is in the change process, having others to turn to can be extremely helpful.

Finally, patients need support in other ways when trying to "get clean" or quit using substances. For example, they may need someone to attend doctors' appointments or meetings (such as Alcoholics Anonymous or Narcotics Anonymous meetings) with them. Supporting the patient also can help family and friends to learn what is happening and how to best help the patient in managing his or her illness and tendency towards using drugs.

Some research shows that certain types of medicines may help people with psychosis who are prone to substance abuse. For example, the newer, atypical antipsychotics may be more beneficial than the older, conventional antipsychotics in helping people to avoid or stop drug abuse. Among the atypical antipsychotic medicines, some research suggests that clozapine may be the most helpful for people with psychosis who are trying to stay clean off drugs.

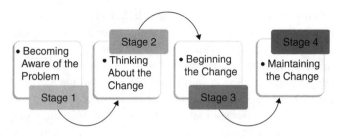

Figure 10.3 Stages of Change

Diet and Exercise

A healthy diet and frequent physical exercise should be part of everyone's life. These two things are necessary for a strong, healthy body and mind. People with an illness especially need to focus on taking care of themselves. For example, if you are diagnosed with diabetes, you may have to start eating differently to control your blood sugar. If you have a broken leg, you may need physical therapy to strengthen your muscles. A change in the way you live is sometimes necessary to feel better and promote long-term health and recovery. One of the best ways to start this new lifestyle is to eat healthier and exercise.

> A change in the way you live is sometimes necessary to feel better and promote long-term health and recovery. One of the best ways to start this new lifestyle is to eat healthier and exercise.

A healthy diet and exercise are especially important for people with psychosis. Overweight/obesity and physical inactivity are two common problems. These problems can eventually lead to medical illnesses like diabetes and heart disease. When going through an episode of psychosis, it is usual to be less active. Symptoms may cause a lack of energy or motivation. In addition, unhealthy eating habits are common among patients, especially in group homes or community centers. Finally, some medicines cause weight gain as a side effect.

These medicines also can cause metabolic side effects. For example, they can sometimes cause elevations in blood glucose and cholesterol levels. Weight gain and metabolic side effects must be carefully monitored by the treatment team because if these occur, they can increase one's risk for future diabetes or heart disease. Some ways in which the doctor may monitor for weight gain and metabolic side effects are discussed in Chapter 6.

People who have or have had psychosis and their caregivers can develop a diet and exercise plan to overcome or prevent weight gain. The plan should include 30 minutes of moderate to intense physical activity (such as brisk walking) at least five days per week. Or, one can do 20 minutes of more vigorous physical activity (such as jogging or running) at least three days per week. People also should try to decrease their intake of sodas, sweets, and other unhealthy snack foods. In addition, they should try to increase the amount of fruits and vegetables in their diet. These are just a few starting ideas for a healthy diet and exercise plan. This plan should be part of the overall treatment plan created with a mental health professional or primary care doctor.

Social Support

For patients to stick with their treatment and to make these necessary lifestyle changes, they will need support from family and friends. Having the support of family and friends is good for one's mental health and physical health. People who have support from others enjoy longer, healthier lives. There are many benefits to having social support from loved ones. These benefits are extremely helpful to people experiencing an episode of psychosis. For example, spending time with others can help to reduce stress. Because stress can trigger symptoms in patients, reducing stress may decrease symptoms or decrease the risk of relapse.

It can be hard to keep relationships with friends or form new relationships with others when going through an episode of psychosis. This is understandable. One reason is that patients have to deal with symptoms that cause problems with socializing. They may have trouble communicating, a lower attention span, or no interest in talking with others. Their ability to feel trusting in others may be impaired. These and other problems can make it hard to get close to others.

It is important to strengthen existing relationships with family and friends. Patients should be encouraged to connect with others. Patients should not be overly protected or restricted. People who have had an episode of psychosis still occasionally become frustrated or angry and need to complain, like everyone else. A supportive environment will allow them to express these emotions without over-reacting. Everyone needs help, especially when going through difficult times. For example, when you have a broken leg or diabetes you may go through periods during which you depend on others. This may be as simple as needing a ride to the doctor.

Patients may think it is hard to find friends who understand and accept them. It is possible; they should not give up. Others may be more open than one might expect. Patients can look to organizations or groups for new connections. Some possible places could be community or church groups. One also could turn to the local chapter of the National Alliance on Mental Illness (NAMI) or Mental Health America (MHA) in the United States, or to similar support organizations in other countries.

> Patients may think it is hard to find friends who understand and accept them. It is possible; they should not give up. Others may be more open than one might expect.

Other people are dealing with these same problems. Others have learned to live with their illness and have full, happy lives through recovery. People who are successfully dealing with a psychotic disorder can help support others with psychosis because they have had their own journey in recovery.

Putting It All Together

A healthy lifestyle is necessary to begin to feel better and move towards recovery. A healthy lifestyle includes not smoking cigarettes, not using drugs, having a healthy diet and exercise routine, and having good social supports. Starting this journey will be difficult, and it may be tempting for someone to turn to substances or away from the help of others.

Mental health professionals can recommend certain therapies, such as nicotine replacement therapy, motivational enhancement therapy, or smoking cessation medicines to help one quit smoking. Treatments for quitting substance use may range from attending regular support meetings, an intensive outpatient program, or even a long-term residential program. Again, discussing options with mental health professionals is important to safely quit using substances.

Other common problems that affect people with psychosis are overweight/obesity and physical inactivity. A healthy diet and regular exercise are important to fight against heart disease, diabetes, and weight gain caused by some medicines. This can be difficult because of a lack of energy or motivation sometimes experienced with an episode of psychosis. However, support from family, friends, mental health professionals, and those who have dealt with psychosis themselves can help the person to succeed. Everyone needs help from others at times, and this is no different for those experiencing psychosis. Keeping up relationships with friends and family and forming new relationships may be difficult. However, supportive groups may be found through church and community groups as well organizations like the National Alliance on Mental Illness (NAMI) or Mental Health America (MHA) in the United States, or similar support organizations in other countries.

Key Chapter Points

- Many people with psychotic disorders smoke cigarettes.
- Cigarette smoking causes the same harm to people with psychosis as it does to anyone else who smokes. In addition, cigarette smoking may interfere with the way the body processes some antipsychotic medicines.
- Some reasons that people abuse substances are to be more social, enhance their pleasure, cope with their symptoms, or try to self-medicate.
- A diet and exercise plan should be included in the patient's treatment plan to deal with problems of weight gain, overweight/obesity, and physical inactivity.
- It may be difficult for people with psychosis to connect with others because of their symptoms. However, social support is important in promoting health.
- Patients will need support from others in order to stick with their treatment and to make necessary lifestyle changes.

Acknowledgments: This chapter was initially developed by Michelle L. Esterberg, MPH, MA. Brian Kirkpatrick, MD, MSPH, served as a collaborator for this chapter.

11 Promoting Recovery

When someone recovers from a physical illness, others often think of him or her as cured. But what about in the field of mental health? Presently, there is no cure for some mental illnesses that cause an episode of psychosis, such as schizophrenia. So, what does it mean for a person with a mental illness like this to recover? One way of thinking about recovery is that instead of people recovering *from* a mental illness, they recover *despite* the mental illness. In other words, people can develop meaningful activities and relationships while learning to manage and live with their mental illness.

Recovery is different from remission. Remission means that the major symptoms, usually positive symptoms like hallucinations and delusions, are no longer active. The goals of remission and recovery go hand in hand. Aiming for remission using medicines (see Chapter 6) and psychosocial treatments (see Chapter 7) is important because recovery is easier when symptoms are under control. But, recovery is a much broader concept, pertaining to one's life goals, rather than to symptom control. Some people experiencing psychosis may appear to recover completely. Others may require ongoing work to improve to the greatest possible level of recovery despite having a long-term illness.

The New Concept of Recovery

The recovery movement is a recent change in thinking about treatment and living with a serious mental illness. Before, to most people, the word *recovery* meant that a patient was symptom-free or improved to some point set by medical professionals. In the new way of thinking, recovery begins by focusing on the person's thoughts and goals about his or her life rather than his or her illness, then moves into helping the individual figure out how he or she fits into his or her own community and larger society. Individuals themselves decide on their personal goals for treatment and recovery instead of mental health professionals deciding for them. Recovery involves an individual reaching his or her goals for independent living, employment, social relationships, and community participation. People with mental illnesses want to be citizens, to participate in shared relationships, and to give something to their communities. Increasing an individual's social skills and ability to function in society is a major part of the recovery process.

In the new concept of recovery, patients are referred to as **consumers**, meaning that they choose which services they will use and how they will use the available services to attain their goals. The goal of the recovery movement is to empower individuals to achieve their fullest potential in life. The recovery philosophy embraces the belief that one can achieve identified and declared life goals when given freedom, support, necessary information, education, and the opportunity to develop skills, jobs, and relationships.

> The goal of the recovery movement is to empower individuals to achieve their fullest potential in life. The recovery philosophy embraces the belief that one can achieve identified and declared life goals when given freedom, support, necessary information, education, and the opportunity to develop skills, jobs, and relationships.

There is no single definition of recovery. People also have different opinions on what type of recovery plan would work best for people with serious mental illnesses. Many in the recovery movement believe that recognizing and honoring the patient as a consumer ultimately translates into the consumer having decision-making power in his or her care. Mental health professionals who agree with the recovery movement assume that this is the best way to help the individual achieve a fulfilled life. As noted earlier, for many patients, recovery is an easier process once symptoms are somewhat under control. Then, they are able to plan the recovery process based on their individual needs.

Principles of Recovery

Some basic ideas about recovery include (also see Figure 11.1):

- **There are many pathways to recovery.** Just as each person's symptoms and life situations are different, each person's journey to recovery will be different as well. Recovery focuses on each individual and what best fits his or her life.
- **Recovery is self-directed and empowering.** Since each person is different, the individual decides what is most important to him or her. These goals are the starting point for recovery plans. For example, if getting a job and finding a place to live independently

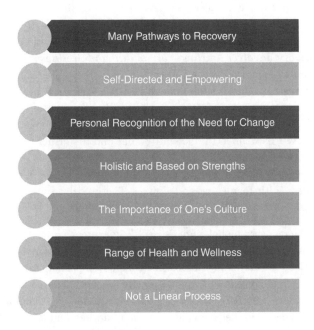

Many Pathways to Recovery

Self-Directed and Empowering

Personal Recognition of the Need for Change

Holistic and Based on Strengths

The Importance of One's Culture

Range of Health and Wellness

Not a Linear Process

Figure 11.1 Principles of Recovery

are most important to that individual, then supported employment and supportive housing are critical services. Because individuals decide themselves, or decide in conjunction with their mental health professional and their family, they can have a strong voice in planning for their future.

- *Recovery requires a personal recognition of the need for change.* Others should not force individuals to change. Only the consumer can decide if a change is necessary for his or her life.

- *Recovery is holistic and based on strengths.* Recovery focuses on mind, body, relationships, activities, and environment. A person has to look at all parts of his or her life when deciding how best to achieve individual goals. Looking at the whole person will help the consumer and others to recognize what issues the person will be dealing with during recovery. Recovery also helps the consumer (and provider) recognize and build on an individual's strengths.

- *One's culture is important in recovery.* When thinking about the whole person, it is necessary to understand his or her cultural background. Understanding a person's culture can clarify an individual's beliefs or attitudes towards his or her illness and recovery.

- *Recovery involves a range of health and wellness.* As noted before, the recovery process does not focus on symptoms. Recovery involves much more, such as health, self-awareness, functioning in desired roles, life satisfaction, self-esteem, and wellness. The nature and quality of the health and wellness of a consumer depends on how it is *defined* by *that* individual and his or her capacity to achieve his or her goals.

- *Recovery is not a linear process.* The recovery process is a lifelong process with many ups and downs. There will be many accomplishments as well as setbacks for the individual.

So, the recovery model emphasizes the consumer's own desires and decisions. This does not go against mental health professionals' recommendations for taking medicines (see Chapter 6), participating in psychosocial treatments (see Chapter 7), or sticking with the treatment plan (see Chapter 8). Rather, the recovery movement aims to strengthen the sharing of decisions between patients, their families, and mental health professionals. Research has shown that medicines and psychosocial treatments are very helpful. This is why mental health professionals often strongly encourage consumers to stick with these treatments. However, in more recent years, patients and their families have shown mental health professionals that they want to be more involved in their own treatment decisions. The recovery movement supports this call for a greater voice in treatment planning and setting goals.

Characteristics of Those in Recovery

Recovery in mental health is a lifelong process. It requires learning, support, courage, and patience. As with any other illness, recovery in a mental illness can have ups and downs. For example, if you have diabetes you may feel worse at times due to your illness; you will undoubtedly have setbacks. On the other hand, there may be times with fewer symptoms. Adhering to a treatment plan will always be a challenge (this is human nature!). The same is true if you have psychosis. To be in a period of recovery, one has to think about both mind and body. It takes more than medicine and therapy.

People in recovery maintain a positive attitude and a sense of hope for their lives. However, they realistically understand that their lives may be different from before. They are aware that it may now be necessary to deal with symptoms and setbacks. Their lives have changed, but they are ready for the challenges ahead.

> People in recovery maintain a positive attitude and a sense of hope for their lives. However, they realistically understand that their lives may be different from before. They are aware that it may now be necessary to deal with symptoms and setbacks.

People in recovery find and capitalize on their strengths and accept themselves. This is often coupled with an ability to take charge of their lives. Maybe they will return to work or school, reconnect with others, or live on their own. More people recover in psychosis than you might think.

While the individual is ultimately in charge of his or her own recovery, having the support of others during this journey is extremely important. It is very helpful to communicate one's needs to family, friends, peers who are also in recovery, health-care providers, and community members. This allows others to offer whatever supports they can and work together with the individual to identify his or her strengths, analyze the existing barriers, and enhance chances of achieving goals.

Putting It All Together

Recovery is a recent social movement in mental health of empowerment and self-determination. It differs from remission because it focuses on more than just symptom control. Instead, the recovery movement focuses on personal goals decided by consumers themselves. Because it is a recent movement, mental health professionals have different opinions on what recovery is. Some basic principles of recovery are that there are many pathways to recovery, it is self-directed and empowering, it requires a personal recognition of the need for change, it is holistic and strengths-based, it considers cultural backgrounds, and it involves a range of health and wellness.

People in recovery will have setbacks. Recovery is a process of learning and patience. One has to think of the whole person—mind and body—to be in a period of recovery. It is an attitude and a way of life. By embracing this empowering philosophy, a large number of people are living in recovery and enjoying their lives. Recovery is possible.

Key Chapter Points

☛ The recovery movement is a recent change in thinking about treatment.

☛ Instead of people recovering *from* psychosis, they recover *despite* psychosis.

☛ Patients are now often referred to as consumers, meaning they choose what services to use and how to use the available services.

☛ The goal of the recovery movement is to empower individuals to achieve their full potential in life.

☛ Having the support of others, including family, friends, peers who are also in recovery, and mental health professionals, during the journey to recovery is extremely helpful to the individual.

☛ To be in a period of recovery, one has to think about both mind and body.

Acknowledgments: This chapter was initially developed by Michelle L. Esterberg, MPH, MA. Robert E. Drake, MD, PhD, and Jacqueline Maus Feldman, MD, served as collaborators for this chapter.

12 Fighting Stigma

Mental health professionals now understand more about mental illnesses than ever before. Effective treatments are available that support many people with mental illnesses living full and productive lives. Despite this and the general public's broader understanding of mental illnesses, negative and incorrect beliefs about these disorders continue. These incorrect beliefs include that mental illnesses are moral failures and that people with mental illnesses are dangerous, incompetent, and unable to function in the community. This can cause persons with mental illnesses and their families to delay seeking treatment in an attempt to avoid being labeled with a mental illness diagnosis. Once diagnosed, they may worry about people finding out and treating them differently. They may experience discrimination in various parts of their lives. This is due to the stigma of mental illness.

Stigma Defined

The traditional definition of **stigma** is a mark of shame that usually lasts forever. Stigma can have negative effects on both the affected person and his or her family. The stigma related to mental illnesses often begins when doctors diagnose the patient with a mental illness. This diagnosis, or label, sometimes links the patient to **stereotypes**, or negative ideas, about people with a mental illness. However, stigma can also begin even before a diagnosis, when the affected person begins to display signs and symptoms of an illness (see Chapter 2). These signs and symptoms (such as talking to oneself or having unusual beliefs) may link the person to negative ideas about those with a mental illness (see Figure 12.1). The stereotypes that society holds about people with mental illnesses are usually wrong. Examples of such ideas are that a person with a mental illness is dangerous, not very intelligent, and unable to work. Other false ideas are that the person has no self-control and will never recover.

Stereotypes can cause others to view people with mental illnesses as different and less human. Not understanding these disorders, others may look down upon or think less of those with a mental illness. As a result, patients and their families may feel that they are less important, or they may feel discriminated against. They also may feel that the stereotypes about those with a mental illness are in some way true. Patients and their families may even feel as though they do not deserve the same rights or respect as people without mental illness. This is called self-stigma. **Self-stigma** occurs when someone with a mental illness holds negative attitudes about mental illnesses. People are generally aware of stigma and, prior to the onset of an illness, they may agree with these negative stereotypes. In this case, a person diagnosed with a mental illness must reconcile those beliefs with their own self-image. **Public stigma** is others' beliefs that lead to instances of discrimination. Public stigma may make people with mental

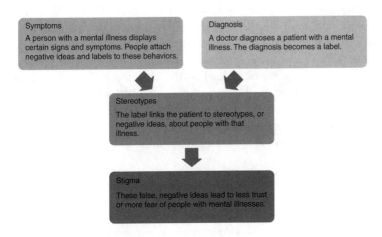

Figure 12.1 The Stigma Process

illnesses worry about what others will think or do. Both self-stigma and expectations and experiences of public stigma could interfere with getting immediate, appropriate treatment.

> Both self-stigma and expectations and experiences of public stigma could interfere with getting immediate, appropriate treatment.

Different mental illnesses carry with them different amounts and types of stigma. For example, depression is not as stigmatized as schizophrenia (see Chapter 3 on What Diagnoses Are Associated with Psychosis?). Unfortunately, and unfairly, schizophrenia and other disorders that cause psychosis are some of the most stigmatized of all mental illnesses. People with psychosis often feel that they do not get the same amount of kindness and understanding about their disease from others compared to people diagnosed with another mental illness or a medical illness.

Stigma and the Media

The media sometimes makes negative ideas even worse by the way they portray a person with a mental illness in movies and on television. For example, some movies, like *Me, Myself & Irene* and *One Flew over the Cuckoo's Nest,* have been criticized for misrepresenting mental illnesses and their treatments in a way that could be damaging to patients and their families. Such negative portrayals cause fear and a lack of trust of people with mental illnesses. It also causes these false ideas to become stronger, leading to even more stigma. More accurate movies and other forms of media—like documentaries, educational books about schizophrenia and other mental illnesses, and Web sites of advocacy groups—may help to decrease stigma. Information about mental illnesses and opportunities to get to know people affected by mental illnesses may also reduce public stigma.

Effects of Stigma

Stigma can have many negative effects. People with psychosis may spend a lot of time on their own (see Chapter 1 on What Is Psychosis?). Although this may be due to negative symptoms, it also may be due to feelings of shame and embarrassment caused by stigma. People with psychosis also may feel as though others do not want to be around them or be friends with them. They may experience discrimination when trying to rent rooms or trying to get and keep a job. They may also worry that people in their community may gossip about them.

Not only do patients feel the effects of stigma, but their families do as well. Generally, those in society react poorly to both patients and their families. People may make unkind comments to them or about them. This can hurt both patients and their families. Often, those in society will react in this way without really knowing about psychosis. Unless people have dealt with psychosis on a personal level, they simply may not understand what the person with the mental illness and the family are experiencing.

> Unless people have dealt with psychosis on a personal level, they simply may not understand what the person with the mental illness and the family are experiencing.

For people with psychosis and their families, the results of stigma may sometimes feel more harmful than the illness itself. Many people do not seek treatment because they are scared of what the label of a mental illness will do to their lives. However, having an untreated mental illness often results in more problems, so getting into and sticking with treatment is important (Chapter 8). Stigma may play a role in how long someone waits before seeking treatment because he or she does not want others to know that something is wrong. In this way, self-stigma or the pain caused by public stigma is sometimes a barrier that people must overcome in order to start treatment. For this reason, it is important for people to be aware of the very negative effect of stigma and work together to fight against it.

Coping with Stigma: Helpful and Harmful Strategies

Because experiencing stigma can be so hurtful, patients and their families use coping strategies to try to deal with it. Some coping strategies can be helpful, but others can make the situation worse.

One helpful coping strategy for families of patients with early psychosis is to bond together to support one another. Family members often have their own negative attitudes about mental illnesses that they must re-evaluate when it becomes a family matter. Unlike society, family members often do not stigmatize a loved one experiencing symptoms of a mental illness, although, unfortunately, this sometimes happens. Families often feel and act very differently towards the patient compared to strangers. They know what their family member is going through and that the negative ideas that society holds are not true. They do not blame the patient for his or her disease. Family members are very important because they are often the ones who bring their loved ones into treatment for the first time. In addition, they are often the ones who encourage and support the patient in sticking with the treatment plan. The next section describes additional helpful ways that families and patients can cope with and fight stigma. But first, know that some attempts to cope with stigma can prove to cause more problems.

Some patients and their families may try to cope with stigma in ways that ultimately are not helpful. For example, they may refuse to accept the diagnosis. This is often a natural reaction to any type of diagnosis—no one wants to have an illness. They also may blame the psychosis on other causes, such as a head injury or the Devil. They might keep the diagnosis a secret since they do not want others looking at them in a different way or as abnormal. Some people might think that mental health problems are embarrassing and hide these problems from others, even from those who can provide care. Hiding problems from some people can sometimes be helpful, but if it causes one to avoid social contacts, it can be harmful. Some might even deny that anything is wrong at all. These types of coping behaviors usually do not work to protect the patient and his or her family from stigma. They also can have a negative effect on the patient's treatment and outcome. Patients and their families can deal with stigma in ways that both support the patient through his or her treatment and fight against stigma.

Successfully Dealing with Stigma

Stigma can be very painful and cause a great deal of shame for people with psychosis and their families. However, it is possible for patients and their families to successfully cope with and fight stigma—and it is a fight to win.

Stigma can be very painful and cause a great deal of shame for people with psychosis and their families. However, it is possible for patients and their families to successfully cope with and fight stigma—and it is a fight to win. Today, there may be less stigma linked to some mental illnesses, like depression. This is because people understand more about the causes of mental illnesses and the effectiveness of treatments. Better treatments are being discovered, so long-term outcomes for patients are getting better. Hopefully, someday the stigma of mental illnesses will disappear. But for now, psychosis, and illnesses that cause psychosis like schizophrenia, remain stigmatized illnesses.

Those with psychosis and their families can take certain steps to help themselves deal with stigma. They can tell others who they trust about the diagnosis. They may not feel comfortable doing so at first because they fear the worst, such as people making fun of them and looking down on them. However, people may in fact treat them with concern and kindness. By breaking their silence, people struggling with a mental illness may gain much-needed support for themselves and their family and no longer have to keep their diagnosis a secret. Deciding who to tell and who not to tell is a personal decision that patients should make after weighing the pros and cons. This can be done in conjunction with a mental health professional.

The patient and his or her family need to remember that they are not alone, even though stigma may cause them to feel alone. There are other people dealing with the same problems. Many people struggle with psychosis, depression, anxiety, substance abuse, and other forms of mental illnesses. It is important to stay in touch with family and friends who can offer support. Being cut off from others can make a person feel even worse and can cause depression and burnout. Patients and their families may want to find out about mental health groups, advocacy, and support groups around the world. We list some of these in Chapter 15 on Seeking More Information.

The fear of stigma must not keep the patient and his or her family from seeking treatment. The earlier the patient gets treatment, the better the chances of recovery. It is very important that patients get into a treatment program and stay in it. Safe antipsychotic medicines (Chapter 6) that work, as well as helpful psychosocial treatments (Chapter 7), are available. Adherence to treatment programs can result in many patients with psychosis enjoying full lives through recovery (Chapter 11).

Finally, if the patient and his or her family feel comfortable enough with the idea, they can share their story with members of their community. By doing so, they may be able to help educate people about the hurt caused by stigmatizing mental illnesses, such as psychosis. Speaking at events can help bring courage to others and educate the public about psychosis. Research has shown that a helpful way to break down the negative ideas that people have about psychosis is to give people the opportunity to get to know a person who has a psychotic disorder. This contact helps people to see the individual behind the label and can reduce the misunderstandings about mental illnesses that lead to stigma.

Even if patients or their families are not ready to speak out in public about what they have gone through, there is still much that they can do. They can speak to close friends or other family members and remind them about the harm in jokes about mental illnesses and negative labels. In addition to speaking out, there are a number of other ways that patients and family members can participate in "stigma-busting" activities of advocacy groups.

Putting It All Together

Despite a better understanding of mental disorders in recent decades, false or inaccurate beliefs still exist in society. A diagnosis of a mental illness sometimes links people with mental illnesses to stereotypes and negative ideas held about these people. These negative ideas can be held by the general public (public stigma) or by the individuals themselves (self-stigma).

There will be times when people say things that hurt. The best way to encourage recovery is to try not to let stigma cause feelings of shame or embarrassment. There will be programs on television or scenes in movies that are unkind. However, other shows and movies (such as *A Beautiful Mind* and *Canvas*) are beginning to portray mental illnesses in a more accurate way. This will hopefully reduce stigma in time. The most important facts are that mental illnesses are medical conditions, that they are no one's fault, and that helpful treatments are available.

People with psychosis also may feel discriminated against when renting rooms or trying to get a job. This is extremely difficult and harmful for patients, families, and friends. It is understandable that some people may not want to enter treatment because they fear the stigma attached to a diagnosis of a mental illness. However, getting into and sticking with treatment is the best way to reduce symptoms and prevent a relapse and hospitalization. Support from family, friends, and advocacy organizations can help the patient to no longer feel alone. If he or she feels comfortable, the patient may choose to tell others or share his or her story with others. This is a personal decision that can only be made after careful thought is given to who he or she would feel comfortable telling.

Mental health is at the beginning of a new age. Now psychosis is not just a disease of the mind; some people are beginning to look at it in the same light as other medical conditions, such as diabetes and heart disease. People with psychosis deserve the same kind of respect, care, and services as people who have other medical conditions. The idea that the individual or the family is to blame and the negative and false ideas linked to psychosis and the illnesses that cause psychosis like schizophrenia will hopefully someday fade away.

The idea that the individual or the family is to blame and the negative and false ideas linked to psychosis and the illnesses that cause psychosis like schizophrenia will hopefully someday fade away.

Key Chapter Points

- ☞ Stigma usually begins with a diagnosis that links the patient to stereotypes, which lead to stigma. It can also begin when people observe symptoms of an untreated mental illness that they do not understand.
- ☞ Low self-esteem, social isolation, shame, and embarrassment are just some of the results of stigma.
- ☞ For people with psychosis and their families, the results of stigma may feel more harmful than the illness itself.
- ☞ People must be aware of the very negative effect of stigma and fight against it.
- ☞ Mental illnesses are medical conditions, they are no one's fault, and helpful treatments are available.
- ☞ Individuals and family members can share their story with others or take part in advocacy activities, which may help others to learn the truth about psychosis and stigma.

Acknowledgments: This chapter was initially developed by Lauren Franz, MBChB, MPH. Amy C. Watson, PhD, served as a collaborator.

13

Reducing Stress, Coping, and Communicating Effectively: Tips for Family Members and Patients

As discussed in previous chapters, psychosis often first begins in late adolescence or young adulthood. Thus, many people who experience a first episode of psychosis live with and rely on their families for support. In addition to providing a place to live and other basic support, families are key in the recovery process because they love and care for the person with the illness and they want to help.

Family members may need to provide emotional support, arrange for treatment, and find new ways to cope with the signs and symptoms of psychosis (see Chapter 2) or other problems that result from the illness. Families are a very important part of the team that is necessary to properly manage psychosis. In fact, now that more effective antipsychotic medicines (see Chapter 6) and psychosocial treatments (see Chapter 7) are available, many people with psychosis often can receive treatment in the community and with their families rather than having extended stays in the hospital. Families play a major role in helping their loved ones manage their illness. As a result, it is vital to create a supportive family environment by reducing stress, coping, and communicating effectively.

This chapter focuses on three essential domains of a supportive family environment: (1) reducing stress, (2) enhancing coping, and (3) ensuring effective communication. First, we begin by defining

> Families play a major role in helping their loved ones manage their illness. As a result, it is vital to create a supportive family environment by reducing stress, coping, and communicating effectively.

stress and the ways that the early stages of psychosis can lead to stress. We discuss three ways to reduce stress in the family as well as three related ways the family can help the patient to reduce stress. Second, we define coping and talk about the importance of coping with a stressful event, like an episode of psychosis in a family member. We offer three ways of coping effectively for family members as well as three ways that patients can practice effective coping. Third, we address the value of good communication and how the symptoms of psychosis can sometimes interfere with productive communication patterns. We then provide eight points of advice for effective communication within the family.

As noted in the Preface, we sometimes use the word *patient* to refer to the individual who has psychosis and who is seeking care from mental health professionals. We realize that this is a medical term and that family members do not think of their loved ones as patients. We use this word for simplicity only, though a more appropriate term would be "loved one dealing with psychosis."

What Is Stress?

The word **stress** describes a feeling of strain, pressure, or tension. Some stress is part of life, and every person and family experiences stress. **Stressors** are events that cause stress. In general, there are two types of stressors: life events and ongoing stressors. **Life events** include things such as becoming ill, experiencing the death of a loved one, going through a divorce, getting married, having a baby, getting a new job, or moving. Some life events are more stressful than others. It is important to remember that whether a life event is positive or negative, it can still be associated with stress. In addition to life events, **ongoing stressors** are a part of everyone's life. Some of these include unwanted or unpleasant household chores, frequent or repeated arguments or conflicts, financial problems, constant criticism, or a chronic illness in a loved one.

Stress can have a wide range of effects on people. These may include physical changes (such as headaches, stomach problems, or heart troubles). Stress can also lead to changes in thinking (such as concentration problems), mood (such as irritability, anxiety, or depression), and behavior (such as restlessness, angry outbursts, or substance use). Learning to manage stress in a healthy way is essential to everyone's physical and mental health.

Stress and the Early Stages of Psychosis

Everyone recognizes that when people become psychotic, they feel stressed. However, it is also normal for family members to feel stress when a person in their family experiences an episode of psychosis. Also, everyone in the family can find the process of learning about the initial evaluation, the diagnosis, and treatment choices to be stressful, overwhelming, and confusing. However, just as one person can pass stress to another, reducing one family member's stress helps to reduce stress for the whole family. So, working together to develop better ways of handling stress strengthens relationships and improves the quality of life for everyone in the family.

Just as the family as a whole will feel stress, the person experiencing the episode of psychosis will obviously feel stress as well. For some people who have experienced psychosis, stress may trigger a relapse (see Chapter 9) and even hospitalization. Thus, it is essential that the family, as well as the patient's mental health professionals, help the patient with ways to reduce stress. Increasing the patient's ability to manage stress helps to decrease his or her risk of symptom relapse.

Ways to Reduce Stress in the Family

There are many ways to reduce stress within the family as a whole; three examples follow.

- *Learn about psychosis.* Families that get educated about psychosis are better able to solve problems and support their loved one. They are better able to reduce stress, cope well, and communicate effectively. This, in turn, can help the patient's illness. Chapter 7 discusses how family interventions, including family psychoeducation and family therapy can be a vital part of the treatment plan. Learning about psychosis requires that the family be comfortable asking questions of

It is essential that the family, as well as the patient's mental health professionals, help the patient with ways to reduce stress. Increasing the patient's ability to manage stress helps to decrease his or her risk of symptom relapse.

health-care providers and/or mental health professionals. Families also can learn about dealing with psychosis and reducing stress by talking to other families who have a loved one with a psychotic disorder.

- *Set reasonable expectations*. The key is to have balance, avoiding extremes. Family members need to set reasonable expectations for themselves. For example, it is not possible to always remain by the patient's side in order to provide support and monitoring. A balance is needed between monitoring and giving the patient enough space to recover and live his or her own life. Family members need to stay engaged in their own lives by making use of support from friends, enjoying hobbies, participating in exercise, and caring for their own physical and mental health.
- *Make time for enjoyable family activities*. Many families do things together. They may enjoy outdoor activities like a picnic, go to the park or lake, attend sporting events, watch a movie, or simply share a family meal together. Family activities may be especially helpful when dealing with serious stress, such as psychosis in a loved one.

Ways for Patients to Reduce Stress

There are many ways that people with psychosis can reduce stress and many things that families can do to help their loved one reduce stress. Examples of things that may help the patient reduce stress, based on the same three general themes listed before for the family as a whole, are described next.

Table 13.1 Ways for Families and
Patients to Reduce Stress

- Learn about psychosis.
- Set reasonable expectations.
- Make time for enjoyable and fulfilling activities.

- *Ask questions about your illness.* Just as families need to learn about psychosis, so does the patient himself or herself. As discussed in Chapter 7 (on Psychosocial Treatments for Early Psychosis), psychoeducation is an essential part of the treatment plan. Like families, patients should feel comfortable asking their mental health professionals questions about psychosis and treatments.
- *Find the right balance.* Just as it is helpful for families to set reasonable expectations, the same is true for the person with a psychotic disorder. Again, the key is to have balance, avoiding extremes. For example, for someone who has recently experienced a psychotic episode, working or going to school full-time may be too demanding at first. But, not working at all may lead to unhappiness because of lack of fulfillment or financial problems. So, working part-time could be fulfilling and provide some financial relief. Reasonable expectations also need to be set for returning to school and for other goals, such as finding a partner and having a child.
- *Enjoy hobbies and recreation.* Just as enjoyable family activities can help reduce stress within the family, hobbies, recreation, and other fulfilling activities are important for patients themselves. For some people, work or school is enjoyable. Others may enjoy being involved in their faith community, volunteer activities, music, exercise or sports, reading, or the arts (art, music, theatre, dance). These, as well as many other activities that bring pleasure, are valuable for reducing one's level of stress.

What Is Coping?

The word **coping** refers to facing and dealing with responsibilities, problems, or difficulties in a successful and calm manner. It is important to keep in mind that one cannot avoid all stressors. Some are just a natural part of trying to fulfill personal goals, a natural part of life. Making a plan to enhance one's coping strategies, or ways of dealing with stress effectively, is very important. Within the family, family members should figure out what type of coping methods each uses and enhance coping strategies to the extent possible. Similar attention to coping strategies is helpful for the patient himself or herself.

How Family Members Can Cope Effectively

Included next are three ways, among many other possibilities, to help families cope with and manage the stress of psychosis in a loved one.

- *Talk and think positively.* The more negatively a person views something, the more stressful it may feel. Many people have self-defeating thoughts when faced with a difficult situation: "This is horrible," "I hate this," or "I won't succeed." Better thoughts to replace these are "I'm going to give it my best try," "While it's not my first choice, I can deal with it," or "It's a challenge, but I can handle it." While changing one's point of view may not get rid of the stressor, it can reduce its impact. Family members can talk and think positively so as not to feel overwhelmed or defeated by their loved one's psychosis. Consistent with the advice to think positively, the recovery model itself focuses on empowerment, optimism, and determination (see Chapter 11).

- *Take care of yourself.* It can be tiring and emotionally draining to care for someone with a mental illness like psychosis. Given the stress of dealing with psychosis in a loved one, it is easy for family members to forget to take time for themselves or even neglect their own needs. In order to be most helpful for the patient, family members must be healthy—both physically and mentally. It is important to take care of oneself through regular exercise, a healthy diet, leisure activities, and good social support. Family members should work on reducing their own stress and seeking care for themselves when it is needed.

> Given the stress of dealing with psychosis in a loved one, it is easy for family members to forget to take time for themselves or even neglect their own needs. In order to be most helpful for the patient, family members must be healthy—both physically and mentally.

- *Embrace your spirituality or other supports.* Faith communities and religious beliefs help many people cope with stress when faced with difficult situations. For some people, prayer and other religious activities may greatly reduce stress. Religious organizations or other community organizations also can provide social support, which can help one to feel less isolated and stressed.

Table 13.2 How Family Members
Can Cope Effectively

- Talk and think positively.
- Take care of yourself.
- Embrace your spirituality or other
  supports.

How the Patient Can Cope Effectively

There are many ways to go about effectively coping with having an illness that causes psychosis; three things that may help the patient cope with the stress of psychosis are described next.

- *Practice relaxation.* A number of techniques can lessen the effects of stress on mental and physical health. Books, classes, recordings, or sessions with trained professionals are all ways to learn these relaxation practices. Some examples include breathing exercises, progressive muscle relaxation, meditation, and yoga. When first learning a technique, it will be necessary to concentrate on doing the steps, but as the steps become familiar it will be easier to relax.
- *Maintain good health habits.* Eating right (a healthy diet) and getting enough sleep can provide the strength to deal with stress. Regular physical exercise can decrease stress, improve sleep, and increase well-being. Almost any physical activity has a positive effect on reducing stress, improving sleep patterns, and lifting mood. It is also important not to smoke cigarettes, not to drink alcohol excessively, and not to use drugs. Maintaining good health habits is not only good for one's long-term health, but it also supports coping with current problems. For more on the importance of good health habits, see Chapter 10 on Staying Healthy.
- *Rely on family, friends, other social supports, and mental health professionals.* Having social supports is good for one's physical and mental health. The support that family members, friends, and others in your community can provide is vital for coping with a serious illness. Additionally, mental health professionals are very knowledgeable not only about the various treatment options, but also about working with people to find their own best ways of reducing stress and coping with the illness.

The Importance of Communication

When people live under strain, no matter the stressor, effective communication often breaks down. Coping with psychosis can be a major strain on everyone involved. It can be especially challenging when the family provides the majority of the care and support for the person with the psychotic disorder. Good communication can lower the amount of stress and conflict in the family. Lower family stress and conflict can help to decrease the possibility of future negative outcomes for family members. It also can reduce the risk of relapse and improve symptoms. Effective communication is helpful in all relationships, including relationships among family members, especially during times of stress.

Table 13.3 How the Patient Can Cope Effectively

- Practice relaxation.
- Maintain good health habits.
- Rely on family, friends, other social supports, and mental health professionals.

Good communication can lower the amount of stress and conflict in the family. Lower family stress and conflict can help to decrease the possibility of future negative outcomes for family members. It also can reduce the risk of relapse and improve symptoms.

Symptoms of Psychosis Can Sometimes Interfere with Communication

Some symptoms of psychosis can make communication between family members and the person who is psychotic difficult at times. Being able to recognize when symptoms are making communication difficult helps family members to respond appropriately. Some reasons why symptoms may make communication difficult are described next.

- ***Positive symptoms can make it difficult for the patient to know what is real and what is not***. Positive symptoms are distracting and can be frightening. Hallucinations can be too difficult to ignore while speaking, and may interfere with communication. The voices may even tell the person experiencing psychosis not to talk or to say things that are inappropriate. Family members should realize that hallucinations are very real to the person experiencing them. The voices are not imagined or made up. Some delusions may cause people to think that anything they say becomes evidence that others can use against them. For example, a person may think that a police agency is recording his or her conversations. Regardless of what the delusion is about, family members should not try to disprove or talk the person out of the delusion. They also should not go along with the delusion given that it does not represent reality and going along with the delusional belief would be dishonest. Paranoia also can interfere with trusting others or feeling safe about expressing thoughts and feelings. It may be helpful to try to empathize with the person who is delusional by taking time to understand what it would feel like to have these troubling experiences.

- *Negative symptoms can make it difficult for family members to know how their relative is feeling.* For example, blunted affect (such as when the face does not show emotion), anhedonia (inability to experience pleasure), and apathy (not caring about what may happen) are often misinterpreted as being lazy or giving up. Not knowing how the person feels can make a conversation very difficult. Family members should realize that these negative symptoms are not under the person's control, but result from the brain dysfunction that underlies the symptoms of psychosis. Sometimes negative symptoms also make it difficult for people to recognize other people's feelings, causing people to miss nonverbal cues, such as facial expression and tone of voice.

- *Disorganization can cause confusion when trying to communicate successfully.* Disorganized thoughts do not make sense logically. The person sounds confused or comes across as confusing. People experiencing this symptom can go so far off topic that they may take a very long time to make a point. At other times, family members may have problems with communication because of unclear, meaningless, or unchanging responses. Being slow or unable to respond to questions also makes communication challenging. It is helpful for family members to be very clear and straight-forward when talking with their loved one with disorganized thoughts. Patience is very important.

- *Cognitive (thinking) problems can cause misunderstandings because of difficulties in concentrating, making decisions, or remembering things.* Someone experiencing psychosis may need more time to think about what someone is saying and to figure out how to respond. Often others give up on them for taking too long or wrongly think the delay is a sign of disinterest.

Advice for Effective Communication within the Family

> Improving communication can improve the overall quality of life for the entire family.

Improving communication can improve the overall quality of life for the entire family. Effective communication helps to reduce relationship problems. It also results in fewer conflicts and unresolved disagreements. This will reduce the level of stress felt by the family and result in fewer emotional problems for all family members. Included next are eight ways to communicate effectively in the family that are sensitive to the challenges posed by psychotic symptoms noted earlier.

- *Be brief and stick to the point.* Keep communications simple and direct, avoiding difficult language. Getting to the point will lessen misunderstandings. Often, people tell all the details of an entire event to help make the story more interesting and to make sure that they do not leave anything out. When talking to someone with psychosis, it is better to make sure to communicate just what one needs to share. For example, instead of saying, "I was going to the bank because I needed some money to buy your prescription, and I ran into your cousin. She has a new haircut and was dressed very professionally. Anyway, I didn't find out what sort of work she's doing now, but she did tell me to say 'hello' to you…," it may be better to say, "I ran into your cousin today, and she asked me to say 'hello' to you."
- *Use "I" statements to communicate feelings.* Verbally expressing both positive and negative feelings lessens the need to guess about what the other person is feeling. This leads to less confusion and tension even when expressing something that is upsetting. One way to do this is by using "I" statements. Instead of referring to someone

else (e.g., "Your uncle thinks you need to wash your hair more often") or asking questions (e.g., "Don't you think you should wash your hair tonight?") it may be better to use "I" statements such as, "I am worried that you aren't washing your hair as often as you used to."

- *Provide positive feedback.* Often, people with a psychotic disorder feel as if they cannot do anything well anymore. It helps to hear that others are proud of them for something or pleased by something that they have done. They will come to understand what their own personal strengths are, instead of focusing only on their limitations. Giving loved ones compliments that are brief and specific encourages them to realize their strengths.
- *Be positive when asking for something.* People who have experienced psychosis may be sensitive to criticism and hostility. Nagging and demanding usually leads to resentment, hurt feelings, and a tendency to not cooperate with requests. It helps to use brief, specific "I" statements in a calm, pleasant voice. For example, instead of saying, "Get to that bedroom of yours already and clean it," or "You're such a slob" it would be better to say, "I would feel better about our home if you would clean your bedroom."
- *Be constructive when upset about something.* Everyone gets upset with others at one point or another. When expressing sadness, frustration, anger, worry, anxiety, or any other negative feelings, it helps to be brief and specific. Remember to not rely solely on facial expressions and tone of voice. Verbally state what is upsetting and then offer suggestions for correcting it or preventing the situation from happening again. Instead of saying, "You're such a hermit," it would be better to say, "I'm worried that you sit in your room all day, and I'd like to sit down and talk about some activities that you might enjoy doing with me or others."
- *Learn how the other person thinks or feels.* Misunderstandings and frustration can occur if a person has negative symptoms and others have to guess about how he or she feels. Instead of guessing, ask. For example, instead of saying, "You don't want to be with me," it would be better to say, "You hardly came out of your room today. I'd feel better if you could tell me how you feel about spending time with me." Family members should verify what the person is saying by rewording what they heard and asking if they understood

Table 13.4 Advice for Effective Communication within the Family

- Be brief and stick to the point.
- Use "I" statements to communicate feelings.
- Provide positive feedback.
- Be positive when asking for something.
- Be constructive when upset about something.
- Learn how the other person thinks or feels.
- Be willing to step back from a stressful situation.
- Compromise.

correctly. For example, if the patient says, "Those people might hurt me," the family member then might say, "So, it sounds like you feel unsafe because of those people you have been thinking a lot about. Is that right? How can I help you to feel safer?"

- ***Be willing to step back from a stressful situation.*** Avoid unnecessarily staying in a stressful or emotionally charged conversation. Taking a break often allows both people to have the chance to calm down so that they can better communicate and solve problems later. It would be helpful to say something like, "Our conversation is stressing me out right now. I'd like to take a break and take a walk so that I can calm down and be better able to talk about this situation later."
- ***Compromise.*** In a compromise, each person usually gets something that he or she wants but also has to give up something. The ultimate goal is to reach a decision that is acceptable to both people. When a compromise occurs, it is a "win-win" situation.

Putting It All Together

Families are a very important source of support for patients who are trying to manage an episode of psychosis. People who have experienced psychosis and their families can work on creating a supportive family environment by reducing stress, coping, and communicating effectively. It is understandable and expected that patients and families would feel stress during an episode of psychosis. However, it is important to reduce stress, which may trigger a relapse or even rehospitalization. Both families and patients can reduce stress by learning about psychosis, setting reasonable expectations, and making time for enjoyable, fulfilling activities.

Because it is impossible to get rid of all stress in one's life, it is important to develop ways to cope with stressors that may occur. Patients and families can use several strategies for coping effectively such as staying positive, taking care of themselves, and seeking support. Stress in a family can sometimes start to break down communication between family members. Certain symptoms can also make communication difficult at times. Good communication can reduce stress, lower conflict, and lower negative outcomes in the family. Certain strategies can help improve communication within the family such as being brief and concise, using "I" statements when communicating feelings, providing positive feedback, being positive when asking for something, being constructive when upset, learning how the other person thinks or feels, being willing to step back when faced with stressful situations, and being willing to compromise.

Mental health professionals may recommend family therapy or family psychoeducation, two valuable psychosocial treatments briefly described in Chapter 7. Research has shown that these family interventions reduce relapse and rehospitalization, improve outcomes, and enhance adjustment. Additionally, family members will benefit from seeking information on psychosis (see Chapter 15), including support that can be gained from organizations such as the National Alliance on Mental Illness (NAMI) and Mental Health America (MHA) in the United States. Similar organizations for patients and families are available in other countries.

Key Chapter Points

☞ Family members are a very important part of the team needed to properly manage psychosis.

☞ It is vital to create a supportive family environment by reducing stress, coping, and communicating effectively.

☞ It is impossible to get rid of all stressors because some are just a natural part of trying to reach personal goals.

☞ Learning to manage stress is important to everyone's mental and physical health.

☞ Working together to develop better ways of handling stress strengthens relationships and improves the quality of life for everyone in the family.

☞ Several simple steps can be taken by family members to work on coping with the symptoms of psychosis in a loved one and by patients to cope with the illness.

☞ Effective communication helps to reduce relationship problems. Effective communication results in fewer conflicts and unresolved disagreements.

Acknowledgments: This chapter was initially developed by Sandra M. Goulding, MPH. Nadine J. Kaslow, PhD, served as a collaborator for this chapter.

14 Finding Specialized Programs for Early Psychosis

Most of the time, people of all different ages and with all sorts of mental illnesses go to the same place to see a doctor, get medicines, or participate in counseling. That is, they go to mental health clinics or the office of a mental health professional that provides treatments for a number of different illnesses. Most young people who have psychosis get their medical care and treatment in a hospital, clinic, or doctor's office. In these places, the doctors and other mental health professionals may have taken special classes about how to help young people with psychosis, but that may not be their only focus. They may see people with other illnesses too.

However, in some places around the world, there are special clinics that are for people in the early stages of psychosis. These types of specialized programs have been developed recently, since the 1990s. These programs have a number of different types of mental health professionals, including psychiatrists, psychologists, nurses, social workers, counselors, and others. In some programs, mental health professionals and doctors in training may rotate through the clinic spending several months at a time training in the clinic. Some programs, like the Early Psychosis Prevention and Intervention Centre (EPPIC) in Melbourne, Victoria, Australia, operate within the framework of a youth health service. Such youth services treat all sorts of mental health issues in young people. Other programs are located primarily in adult mental health facilities.

Such programs may offer classes or group meetings just for people who recently developed psychosis and other classes or group meetings especially for the families of these young people. Typically, these programs provide someone with 2–3 years of treatment. They usually do a full evaluation of the patient every few months and keep track of how he or she is doing. If the patient needs more care afterwards, they help him or her find another program for longer-term care. In this chapter, we list some of these clinics located in various parts of the world and describe what these specialized early psychosis programs provide.

Where Are Special Programs for Early Psychosis?

Programs for people who have recently had their first episode of psychosis are not available everywhere. These programs are usually in big cities, where there are more young people with psychosis in one place. There are programs just for early psychosis in many countries around the world. In this chapter, we focus on those in several English-speaking countries, including Australia, Canada, Ireland, the United Kingdom, and the United States. It is common for these programs to be near a large university. Many times, they not only offer medical care to patients, but they also do research to help mental health professionals develop even better treatment programs.

What Do Special Programs for Early Psychosis Provide?

Not all programs for people with a first episode of psychosis are the same. Some programs are in big hospitals and others are in smaller clinics. While some programs may admit patients overnight (hospitalization), others may not. However, despite some differences, most of these specialized early psychosis program have a number of things in common.

As mentioned earlier, many of these programs provide treatment to patients for about 2–3 years after they start treatment for psychosis for the first time. Most programs provide a combination of services, including medicines, therapy, classes, groups, case management, mobile crisis teams, and community outreach. Every program in Table 14.1 does not necessarily offer all of these services. However, they usually do provide some combination of different treatments. The

Table 14.1 Specialized Early Psychosis Programs

Australia		
Location	**Name of the Program**	**Web site or City/State/Province/Country**
Dandenong, Victoria	Recovery and Prevention of Psychosis Service (RAPPS)	Dandenong, Victoria, Australia
Noarlunga Centre, South Australia	Noarlunga Early Psychosis Program	Noarlunga, Adelaide, South Australia,
Newcomb, Victoria	Barwon Health Early Intervention Service	http://www.barwonhealth.org.au/services/mentalhealth/Service,documentId,604.aspx
Parkville, Victoria	Early Psychosis Prevention and Intervention Centre (EPPIC)	http://www.eppic.org.au
Taree, New South Wales	Mid North Coast Early Psychosis Program	Taree, New South Wales, Australia

Canada		
Location	**Name of the Program**	**Web site or City/State/Province/Country**
Calgary, Alberta	The Early Psychosis Treatment Program	http://www.calgaryhealthregion.ca/mh/sites/EPTP/epp/index.htm
Halifax, Nova Scotia	The Nova Scotia Early Psychosis Program (NSEPP)	http://earlypsychosis.medicine.dal.ca
Hamilton, Ontario	The Cleghorn Program	http://www.stjoes.ca/default.asp?action=article&ID=365
London, Ontario	Prevention and Early Intervention Program for Psychosis (PEPP-London)	http://www.pepp.ca
Montreal, Quebec	Prevention and Early Intervention Program for Psychoses (PEPP-Montreal)	http://www.douglas.qc.ca/clinical-services/adults/specialized/pepp.asp?l=e
North Bay, Ontario	Regional Early Intervention in Psychosis Program	http://www.nemhc.on.ca/programs-services/regional-specialized/early-intervention-e.aspx
Ottawa, Ontario	First Episode Psychosis Program	http://www.ottawahospital.on.ca/patient/visit/clinics/psychosis-e.asp
Penticton, British Columbia	South Okanagan Early Psychosis Intervention Program	Penticton , British Columbia, Canada
Toronto, Ontario	Toronto First Episode Psychosis Program (FEPP)	http://www.camh.net/About_CAMH/Guide_to_CAMH/Mental_Health_Programs/Schizophrenia_Program/guide_first_episode_program.html
Vancouver, British Columbia	HOPE: Helping Overcome Psychosis Early	http://www.hopevancouver.com
White Rock, British Columbia	The Early Psychosis Intervention (EPI) Program	http://www.earlypsychosisintervention.ca/epi

(continued)

Table 14.1 Continued

Ireland

Location	Name of the Program	Web site or City/State/Province/Country
Dublin	Dublin and East Treatment and Early Care Team (DETECT)	http://www.detect.ie
South Dublin	Detection, Education and Local Team Assessment (DELTA)	http://www.deltaproject.ie

New Zealand

Location	Name of the Program	Web site or City/State/Province/Country
Christchurch, New Zealand	Totara House Early Intervention in Psychosis Service	http://www.cdhb.govt.nz/totara/totara.htm

Norway

Location	Name of the Program	Web site or City/State/Province/Country
Stavanger	Early Treatment and Intervention in Psychosis (TIPS)	http://www.tips-info.com

Singapore

Location	Name of the Program	Web site or City/State/Province/Country
Singapore	Early Psychosis Intervention Program (EPIP)	http://www.epip.org.sg

United Kingdom

Location	Name of the Program	Web site or City/State/Province/Country
Epsom, Surrey	Early Intervention in Psychosis (EIIP)	Epsom ,Surrey, England
Fulbourn, Cambridge	CAMEO	www.cameo.nhs.uk
London	Lambeth Early Onset (LEO) Team	http://www.slam.nhs.uk/services/servicedetail.aspx?dir=5&id=506

United States

Location	Name of the Program	Web site or City/State/Province/Country
California		
Los Angeles, California	AfterCare Research Program	http://www.schizophrenia.ucla.edu/aftercare/
Sacramento, California	Early Diagnosis and Preventive Treatment of Psychotic Illness	http://earlypsychosis.ucdavis.edu/home/index.php

(continued)

Table 14.1 Continued

Location	Name of the Program	Web site or City/State/Province/Country
Connecticut		
New Haven, Connecticut	Specialized Treatment Early in Psychosis (STEP) Program	http://specializedtreat-mentearlyinpsychosi.com
Hartford, Connecticut	POTENTIAL Clinic	http://www.instituteofliving.org/Programs/Schizophrenia/potential.htm
Illinois		
Chicago, Illinois	First Episode Psychosis Clinic	http://ccm.psych.uic.edu/NeedDoctor/FEPClinic/FEPClinic.aspx
Massachusetts		
Boston, Massachusetts	First Episode and Early Psychosis Program (FEPP)	http://www.massgeneral.org/allpsych/Schizophrenia/scz_care_treatment-1st-epi.html
Boston, Massachusetts	Prevention and Recovery in Early Psychosis: The PREP Program	http://www.massmental-healthcenter.org/clinicalservices/programsandservices-prep.htm
Michigan		
Detroit, Michigan	Services for the Treatment in Early Psychoses (STEP)	http://www.med.wayne.edu/psychiatry/UPG%20Website/adult/step.html
North Carolina		
Chapel Hill, North Carolinav	OASIS (Outreach and Support Intervention Services)	http://www.med.unc.edu/wrkunits/2depts/psych/clinicalservices/oasis.htm
Oregon		
Salem, Oregon	Early Assessment and Support Team (EAST)	http://www.eastcommunity.org/home/ec1/smartlist_61/about_east.html

idea behind programs that have more than one part is that the different pieces work best if provided together. We describe each of these seven services in the following pages. Researchers now believe that providing **phase-specific care** is best for patients with a first episode of psychosis. This means that the treatment plan for each individual patient is tailored to his or her own needs, depending on the kinds of symptoms present, how severe the symptoms are, and the types of other problems going on in the patient's life.

> Most programs provide a combination of treatments, including medicines, therapy, classes, groups, case management, community outreach, and mobile teams.... The idea behind programs that have more than one part is that the different pieces work best if provided together.

Case Management

Case management is an important part of many programs designed especially for young people with psychosis. Case management is a treatment service in which one person is in charge of checking in with the patient on a regular basis and making sure that he or she has all the services needed. Case managers are usually nurses, social workers, or other health professionals who help patients to coordinate services. They can work alone or in teams. Case managers in many programs call or visit the patient at least once a week. They ask how the person is doing and if he or she needs anything. They also help people find and sign up for things like classes, groups, and programs. The purpose is to help someone with psychosis live more independently and to help families as well. The case manager usually talks to the patient's other mental health professionals about any new symptoms or issues that come up. In this way, the case manager helps to make sure that the program is providing the patient with as many helpful treatments and services as are available.

Medicines

Programs for people with a first episode of psychosis always provide an evaluation by a psychiatrist who can prescribe medicines to patients. Most programs for patients with early psychosis start patients on a low dosage of an atypical antipsychotic medicine (see Chapter 6 on Medicines Used to Treat Psychosis).

Psychosocial Treatments

In addition to antipsychotic medicines, most programs for people with a first episode of psychosis offer psychosocial treatments. These treatments aim to help the person with symptoms of psychosis and with other problems that sometimes happen as a result of psychosis. For example, psychosocial treatments may focus on depression, substance abuse, unemployment, and relationship difficulties. Psychosocial treatments can be helpful, especially in combination with medicines, for people who are recovering from psychosis.

Psychosocial treatments often include individual therapy sessions, classes, or group sessions (see Chapter 7 on Psychosocial Treatments for Early Psychosis). Cognitive-behavioral therapy, which helps people examine and improve their thoughts and actions, is often the basis for individual therapy sessions. In addition, programs may provide other forms of individual counseling or therapy. Some programs also offer classes on topics such as social skills and employment. These classes help patients to catch up on opportunities that may have been lost during the early stages of psychosis, like learning social skills or job skills. This helps patients to get back to spending time with friends and going to work, which is a part of recovery and leading a fulfilling life. Some programs offer classes about psychosis. These classes may be for people with psychosis themselves, but it is also very common for programs to provide classes like this for family members. These psychoeducation groups for patients, as well as family psychoeducation for a single family or in multi-family groups, are discussed in Chapter 7. Finally, many programs designed for young people with early psychosis include support groups. Like classes, programs may provide support groups to patients, families, or patients and families together.

Mobile Crisis Teams

Many specialized programs for young people with a first episode of psychosis work with local **mobile crisis teams**. These mobile teams usually include several people who go to talk with someone who may have psychosis in his or her school, home, or wherever else he or she may be. Mobile teams sometimes also work closely with hotlines. This is so that they can get a phone call from a doctor, a school administrator, or a family member who is worried about someone. They then try to go and meet with that person who may benefit from treatment.

The mobile team can do an evaluation without always having to take the person to a health-care setting. They can talk to that person about what is going on and what the options are. If someone is a danger to himself or herself or others, they may take that person to the hospital for treatment, even if he or she does not want to go (see Chapter 5 on The Initial Evaluation of Psychosis). If hospitalization is not necessary, the mobile crisis team makes recommendations and lets the individual and his or her family know about available services.

Sometimes mobile teams work with police officers. Unfortunately, police are sometimes the first people to bring a young person with psychosis in to care. This can be a frightening experience for someone with psychosis, and it may be a bad start to his or her care. Mobile teams are set up in some cities so that when the police are notified of someone who may be psychotic, a mental health professional can go with an officer to talk to that person and see if he or she needs medical care. The mobile units sometimes go to people in a regular car (rather than a police car or ambulance).

Community Outreach

Many programs for young people with psychosis provide community outreach to educate people about psychosis and to encourage people to get treatment early. Often, they do two kinds of community outreach at the same time. First, they do general outreach to everyone. The community outreach program may make radio announcements or put posters in public places like bus stations. Most programs also have user-friendly Web sites where the public can find much information. We list some of these Web sites in Tables 14.1 and 14.2. Sometimes people who have had psychosis or their families help to educate others about psychosis. The purpose of this kind of public education is usually to teach everyone about the early signs and symptoms of psychosis (see Chapter 2), to try to reduce stigma (see Chapter 12), and to let everyone know that evaluation and treatment are readily available.

The second kind of community outreach focuses more on doctors, school counselors, and other people who may meet someone with early psychosis in the community. In these educational programs for doctors, school counselors, and other professionals, the community outreach program sends flyers and makes phone calls to make sure that these individuals know about the available services.

Programs like this can really help! Researchers have found that people come to clinics earlier when there are outreach campaigns in a community. This is important because the earlier you evaluate and treat someone with psychosis, the better they tend to do in the long term. Some groups of researchers are working to reduce delays in seeking treatment in order to make it easier for patients and families to enter evaluation and treatment for the first time. For example, research from Norway indicates that community outreach programs, both to the general public and to doctors and school counselors, help patients enter treatment earlier, which then helps them to do better.

Programs like this can really help! Researchers have found that people come to clinics earlier when there are outreach campaigns in a community. This is important because the earlier you evaluate and treat someone with psychosis, the better they tend to do in the long-term.

Treatments during the Prodromal Phase

In some places, specialized clinics and treatment programs have been developed to try to identify and help people who are about to develop psychosis, before the psychosis begins. Such programs do this by providing services to people who appear to be at a high risk for developing psychosis. These people have the same types of symptoms seen in the prodromal phase of a psychotic disorder. Usually, before someone has psychosis for the first time, he or she gradually develops milder symptoms, such as social withdrawal, unusual ideas, or seeing things in shadows (see Chapter 9 on Early Warning Signs and Preventing a Relapse). Not everyone who has these types of milder symptoms will go on to develop psychosis, but they have symptoms that put them at risk for developing psychosis. For those who do develop psychosis, this period of initial symptoms is called the prodrome, or prodromal phase (see Chapter 1 on What Is Psychosis?).

Treatment programs for people in the prodromal stage can be very helpful. They usually consist of psychosocial treatments, similar to

Table 14.2 Specialized Prodrome Clinics

Australia

Location	Name of the Program	Web site or City/State/Province/Country
Dandenong, Victoria	Recovery and Prevention of Psychosis Service (RAPPS)	Dandenong, Victoria, Australia
Parkville, Victoria	The PACE Clinic	http://www.orygen.org.au/ contentPage .asp?pageCode=PACE

Canada

Location	Name of the Program	Web site or City/State/Province/Country
Toronto, Ontario	PRIME (Prevention through Risk Identification, Management and Education) Clinic	www.camh.net/prime_clinic

Norway

Location	Name of the Program	Web site or City/State/Province/Country
Stavanger	The TOPP (early Treatment Of Pre-Psychosis) Clinic	http://www.tips-info.com

United Kingdom

Location	Name of the Program	Web site or City/State/Province/Country
Epsom, Surrey	Early Intervention in Psychosis (EIIP)	Epsom, Surrey, England
London	Outreach and Support in South London (OASIS)	http://www.slam.nhs.uk/services/ servicedetail.aspx?dir=5&id=939

United States

Location	Name of the Program	Web site or City/State/Province/Country
California		
Los Angeles, California	The Staglin Music Festival Center for the Assessment and Prevention of Prodromal States (CAPPS)	http://www.capps.ucla.edu
Sacramento, California	EDAPT (Early Diagnosis and Preventive Treatment)	http://earlypsychosis.ucdavis.edu/ home/index.php http://preventmentalilllness.ucdavis. edu/web-content/ about_edapt_sac. html

(continued)

Table 14.2 Continued

Location	Name of the Program	Web site or City/State/Province/Country
San Francisco, California	PART (Prodrome Assessment Research and Treatment) Program	http://psych.ucsf.edu/research.aspx?id=1328
Connecticut		
New Haven and Hartford, Connecticut	PRIME (Prevention through Risk Identification, Management and Education)	http://www.med.yale.edu/psych/clinics/ prime/pintro.html
Maine		
Portland, Maine	The Portland Identification and Early Referral (PIER) program	http://www.preventmentalillness.org /pier_home.html
Michigan		
Ypsilanti, Michigan	Michigan Prevents Prodromal Progression (M3P)	http://www.preventmentalillnessmi.org /aboutm3p.html
Missouri		
St. Louis, Missouri	The Conte Center First Contact Program	http://www.conte.wustl.edu/psych/conteweb.nsf/WV/D348285BE1257F77862571110060A98A?OpenDocument
New York		
New York , New York	The Center of Prevention and Evaluation (COPE)	http://cumc.columbia.edu/dept/pi /research/clinics/pc.html
Queens, New York	The Recognition and Prevention Program (RAP)	http://www.rapprogram.org/aboutRAP.html
North Carolina		
Chapel Hill, North Carolina	PRIME (Prevention through Risk Identification, Management and Education)	http://www.prime.unc.edu/

the ones listed earlier and explained more thoroughly in Chapter 7. In some cases, doctors in these specialized prodrome clinics prescribe a medicine for someone in the prodromal stage. This can decrease the severity of the prodromal symptoms and perhaps even keep people from getting full-blown psychosis (or delay the onset of psychosis for some time). However, the doctor will very carefully weigh the benefits and the risks of taking medicine at this early stage and will discuss the benefits and risks with the patient and his or her family. If a medicine is started, the patient will be carefully monitored for the development of any side effects. Also, mental health professionals in these specialized prodrome clinics help people to get treatment as early as possible if they do develop an episode of psychosis. Table 14.2 lists some of these specialized clinics for adolescents and others who may be in the prodromal phase of psychosis.

Putting It All Together

If you or someone you know is experiencing psychosis for the first time you may find a special program for early or first-episode psychosis to be particularly helpful. This is because such programs have specially trained mental health professionals, provide the best-proven treatments, and conduct research. We have listed some of the programs like this that are available, but there are more programs not on this list. In addition to these programs, there are also programs that treat people who are at high risk for developing psychosis or who may be in the prodromal phase. We have also listed some of these programs, but more are available.

If you are looking for a program, you may be able to find one through an Internet search or by asking a mental health professional in your local area. The programs listed here may also be able to direct you to a similar program near you. You can find more advice on how to get the information you need in Chapter 15 on Seeking More Information. If there is no special program for early psychosis in your area, you could also look for a treatment facility with doctors who specialize in psychosis or schizophrenia, or a more general program that has some of the same services listed earlier.

Key Chapter Points

☛ Most young people who have psychosis get their medical care and treatment in a hospital, clinic, or doctor's office that does not focus only on first-episode psychosis. However, in some places around the world, there are special clinics designed for people having a first episode of psychosis.

☛ Most specialized programs provide a combination of services, including medicines, therapy, classes, groups, case management, mobile crisis teams, and community outreach.

☛ Case management consists of one person who is in charge of checking in with the patient on a regular basis and making sure that he or she has all the services needed.

☛ Mobile crisis teams usually consist of several people who go to a school, home, or other sites to talk with someone who may have psychosis or another mental illness or be in a crisis situation.

☛ Many programs for young people with psychosis provide community outreach to educate people about psychosis and to encourage people to get treatment early.

☛ In some places, there are clinics and treatment programs that try to identify people at risk for developing psychosis and help them before psychosis even starts, during the prodromal phase of a psychotic disorder.

Acknowledgments: This chapter was initially developed by Claire E. Ramsay, MPH. Jane Edwards, PhD, Inge Joa, MHS, RN, and Tor K. Larsen, MD, PhD, served as collaborators for this chapter.

15 Seeking More Information

As we have discussed in previous chapters, it is very important for people with psychosis and their family members to learn about psychosis and effective treatments. This sort of learning is an important step towards recovery (see Chapter 11) and preventing a relapse (see Chapter 9). However, seeking information to better understand psychosis can be frustrating at times. The amount of information received from mental health professionals and other sources can be overwhelming. However, aside from this book, very few books focus on first-episode psychosis. When searching the Internet, it is difficult at times to tell the difference between Web sites with correct and helpful information from those that contain opinions and confusing information. This chapter describes the benefits of educating yourself about psychosis and then describes different resources that are available.

Psychoeducation

As discussed in Chapter 7 on Psychosocial Treatments for Early Psychosis, **psychoeducation** is a type of education that focuses on the topic of mental illnesses. The goal of psychoeducation is to help individuals with a mental illness, and their family members, better understand the illness. If a person understands his or her illness, then he or she will be able to deal with it more successfully. Psychoeducation, for both patients and their families, is an effective form of treatment in itself and an important step in preventing relapse and hospitalization.

Research has shown that those who receive psychoeducation are less likely to have a relapse and enter the hospital compared to those who do not receive psychoeducation.

Talking to Your Mental Health Professional

The patient's mental health professional is one of the best sources of information. Do not be afraid to ask him or her to explain more if some piece of information is unclear. Another good idea is to bring a list of questions with you when you meet with the mental health professional to make sure that you leave the appointment with all of your questions answered. Asking questions and getting answers helps you become confident that you understand the next steps. Worksheets provided in Chapters 2 and 9 will help you keep track of information that may be important to share with the mental health professional. Worksheets provided in Chapters 6 and 7 will help you keep track of important information that you receive at the appointment.

> Your mental health professional is one of your best sources of information. Do not be afraid to ask him or her to explain more if some piece of information is unclear.

It is normal to feel overwhelmed by all of the information you are receiving and to not know where to start when asking questions. One way to start is to follow the "Ask Me 3" guidelines recommended to encourage clear communication between patients and health-care providers (http://www.npsf.org/askme3):

1. What is my main problem?
2. What do I need to do?
3. Why is it important for me to do this?

Information on Psychosis from Books and Magazines

Getting extra information from sources like books and magazines also can be helpful. Using these sources allows people to educate themselves at their own pace. However, at this time most books focus on specific diagnoses, such as schizophrenia or bipolar disorder, instead

Table 15.1 Books and Magazines on Schizophrenia

Title	Author	Year	Publisher
100 questions and answers about schizophrenia: Painful minds.	Lynn E. Delisi	2006	Jones and Bartlett
The complete family guide to schizophrenia.	Kim T. Mueser & Susan Gingerich	2006	The Guilford Press
Coping with schizophrenia: A guide for families.	Kim T. Mueser & Susan Gingerich	1994	New Harbinger
Coping with schizophrenia: A guide for patients, families, and caregivers.	Steven Jones & Peter Hayward	2004	Oneworld
Diagnosis schizophrenia.	Rachel Miller & Susan E. Mason	2002	Columbia University Press
Getting your life back together when you have schizophrenia.	Roberta Temes	2002	New Harbinger
How to live with schizophrenia.	Abram Hoffer & Humphrey Osmond	1992	Carol Publishing Group
If your adolescent has schizophrenia: An essential resource for parents.	Raquel E. Gur & Ann Braden Johnson	2006	Oxford University Press
Learning about schizophrenia: Rays of hope. A reference manual for families and caregivers (3rd ed.).	Schizophrenia Society of Canada	2003	Schizophrenia Society of Canada
Schizophrenia (2nd ed.).	Sophia Frangou & Robin M. Murray,	2000	Martin Duntz
Schizophrenia Digest.	Kathryn Smithyman, Editor-in-Chief	Quarterly publication www.szdigest.com	Magpie Media, Inc.
Schizophrenia: Straight talk for family and friends.	Maryellen Walsh	1985	William Morrow and Company
Surviving schizophrenia: A manual for families, consumers, and providers (4th ed.).	E. Fuller Torrey	2001	Harper Collins

of first-episode psychosis more generally. Several books on schizophrenia provide excellent information for patients and families. Table 15.1 lists a number of these books.

Web Sites with Information on Psychosis

Another way to get more information about psychosis and other mental illnesses is from the Internet. Some relevant Web sites are from organizations that provide support to those with mental illnesses and their families. Examples of such organizations in the United States are the National Alliance on Mental Illness (NAMI) and Mental Health America (MHA). These Web sites offer information on psychosis as well as on coping with mental illnesses. One can find contact information for local chapters of those organizations on the Web sites listed in Table 15.2. Similar support organizations exist around the world.

Another way to get more information about psychosis and other mental illnesses is from the Internet. Some relevant Web sites are from organizations that provide support to those with mental illnesses and their families.

Other Web sites listed in Table 15.2 are from research programs and specialized first-episode clinics such as ORYGEN Youth Health, PEPP, and TIPS (see Chapter 14 on Finding Specialized Programs for Early Psychosis). These Web sites provide information on psychosis as well as research projects that individuals can participate in and available treatment programs.

When trying to figure out which Web sites contain correct and helpful information, Web addresses that end in domain names of .gov, .org, and .edu are a good place to start. Different divisions of government, not-for-profit organizations, or universities usually sponsor these Web sites. Other Web sites also may contain useful information. Table 15.2 lists some Web sites that provide useful information on psychosis.

Putting It All Together

Valuable information about psychosis is available for patients and families. This information will help patients and their families to deal with psychosis successfully and to live a full life. Knowledge and a better understanding of psychosis is important in preventing relapse and rehospitalization. While information is available through books, magazines and Web sites, mental health professionals also are excellent sources of information. It is important to talk with the mental health professional and clear up any questions or concerns that you may have.

Table 15.2 Web Sites with Helpful Information on Psychosis

Web site	Web Address	Information Provided
Canadian Mental Health Association (CMHA)	www.cmha.ca	Provides information on topics such as mental health, mental illnesses, available support, and advocacy opportunities.
Early Treatment and Intervention in Psychosis (TIPS)	www.tips-info.com	Available in English. Provides information on psychosis, research projects, receiving help, as well as useful links.
International Early Psychosis Association	www.iepa.org.au	Provides information on current international research and a list of available early psychosis services.
Mental Health America (MHA)	www.nmha.org	Provides information on topics such as mental health, disorders, treatment, receiving help, and advocacy opportunities.
Mental Health Association	www.mentalhealth. asn.au	Provides links to state-specific Web sites in Australia. These Web sites provide information on available services, factsheets on specific mental illnesses, and links to related Web sites.
Mental Health First Aid (MHFA)	www.mhfa.com.au	Provides a list of MHFA courses, first aid strategies for a number of mental health problems, guidelines, newsletters, and useful links.
National Alliance on Mental Illness (NAMI)	www.nami.org	Provides information on topics such as mental illnesses, medicine, and research as well as support options and advocacy opportunities.
National Institute of Mental Health (NIMH)	http://www.nimh. nih.gov/health/topics/ schizophrenia/index. shtm	Provides information on specific disorders and outreach programs as well as additional resources and links to related Web sites.
ORYGEN Youth Health	www.orygen.org.au	Provides fact sheets, online resources, links to additional Web sites, and information on services.
Prevention and Early Intervention Program for Psychoses (PEPP)	www.pepp.ca	Provides information on services and links to related sites.
ReThink	www.rethink.org	Provides information about mental illnesses, living with mental illnesses, and available services.
SAMHSA'S National Mental Health Information Center	http://mentalhealth. samhsa.gov	Provides publications, information on mental health topics, programs, and other available resources.

Key Chapter Points

☛ The goal of psychoeducation is to help individuals with a mental illness, and their family members, better understand the illness.

☛ Asking the mental health professional questions and getting answers helps you become confident that you understand the next steps.

☛ Getting extra information from sources like books also can be helpful. Using books or Web sites to find information allows people to educate themselves at their own pace.

☛ Organizations such as the National Alliance on Mental Illness (NAMI) and Mental Health America (MHA) provide support to those with mental illnesses and their families.

☛ When trying to figure out which Web sites contain correct and helpful information, Web addresses that end in domain names of .gov, .org, and .edu are a good place to start, although other Web sites also may contain useful information.

16 Understanding Mental Health First Aid for Psychosis

Throughout this guide, we have tried to explain all parts of a first episode of psychosis in a detailed way. But what happens if you know someone who may be experiencing an episode of psychosis and you have to act fast or help them get into treatment? This last chapter includes advice on how to provide mental health "first aid" to those who may be experiencing an episode of psychosis. These guidelines were developed by and reprinted here with permission from Professor Anthony Jorm and Ms. Betty Kitchener from the University of Melbourne and ORYGEN Research Centre in Melbourne, Victoria, Australia. As a result of an extensive process, they are based on the agreement of a panel of patients, family members, and mental health professionals from Australia, Canada, New Zealand, the United Kingdom, and the United States. For more information on their Mental Health First Aid program, please visit www.mhfa.com.au. The remainder of this chapter is organized around nine questions that are addressed to help people who may need to provide "first aid" to someone experiencing psychosis.

Purpose of These Guidelines

The purpose of these guidelines is to help members of the public to provide first aid to someone who may be experiencing psychosis. The role of the first aider is to assist the person until he or she receives appropriate professional help or the crisis resolves.

How to Use These Guidelines

These guidelines are a general set of recommendations about how you can help someone who may be experiencing psychosis. Each individual is unique, and it is important to tailor your support to that person's needs. So, these recommendations will not be appropriate for every person who may have psychosis.

How Do I Know If Someone Is Experiencing Psychosis?

It is important to learn about the early warning signs of psychosis (see Chapter 9) and the symptoms of psychosis (see Chapter 2) so that you can recognize when someone may be developing psychosis. Although some of these signs may not be very dramatic on their own, when you consider them together, they may suggest that something is not quite right. It is important not to ignore or dismiss such warning signs or symptoms, even if they appear gradually and are unclear. Do not assume that the person is just going through a phase or misusing alcohol or other drugs, or that the symptoms will go away on their own.

> It is important not to ignore or dismiss warning signs or symptoms, even if they appear gradually and are unclear. Do not assume that the person is just going through a phase or misusing alcohol or other drugs, or that the symptoms will go away on their own.

You should be aware that the signs and/or symptoms of psychosis may vary from person to person and can change over time. You should also consider the spiritual and cultural context of the person's behaviors, because what one culture thinks is a symptom of psychosis may be normal in another culture.

How Should I Approach Someone Who May Be Experiencing Psychotic Symptoms?

People developing a psychotic disorder often will not reach out for help. Someone who is experiencing profound and frightening changes such as psychotic symptoms often will try to keep them a secret. If you are concerned about someone, approach the person in a caring and nonjudgmental way to discuss your concern. The person you are trying to help might not trust you or might be afraid that you will view him or her as "different," and therefore may not be open with you. If possible, you should approach the person privately about his or her experiences in a place that is free of distraction.

Try to tailor your approach and interaction to the way the person is behaving. For example, if the person is suspicious and avoiding eye contact, be sensitive to this and give the person the space he or she needs. Do not touch the person without his or her permission. You should state the specific behaviors you are concerned about and should not guess about the person's diagnosis. It is important to allow the person to talk about his or her experiences and beliefs if he or she wants to. When possible, let the person set the pace and style of the interaction. You should recognize that the individual may be frightened by his or her thoughts and feelings. Ask the person about what will help him or her to feel safe and in control. Reassure the individual that you are there to help and support him or her and that you want to keep him or her safe. If possible, offer the person choices of how you can help so that he or she is in control. Express a message of hope by assuring the individual that help is available and things can get better.

If the person is unwilling to talk with you, do not try to force him or her to talk about his or her experiences. Instead, let him or her know that you will be available if he or she would like to talk in the future.

How Can I Be Supportive?

Treat the person with respect. You should try to understand how the person feels about his or her beliefs and experiences without stating any judgments about those beliefs and experiences. The person may be behaving and talking differently due to psychotic symptoms. He or she also may find it difficult to tell what is real from what is not real. You should avoid confronting the person with criticism or blame. Understand the symptoms for what they are and try not to take them personally. Do not use sarcasm, and try to avoid using patronizing statements. It is important that you are honest when interacting with the person. Do not make any promises that you cannot keep.

How Do I Deal with Delusions and Hallucinations?

It is important to recognize that the delusions and hallucinations are very real to the person. You should not dismiss, minimize, or argue with the person about his or her delusions or hallucinations. Similarly, do not act alarmed, horrified, or embarrassed by the person's delusions or hallucinations. You should not laugh at the person's symptoms of psychosis. If the person displays paranoid behavior, do not encourage or inflame the person's paranoia.

> It is important to recognize that the delusions and hallucinations are very real to the person.

How Do I Deal with Communication Difficulties?

People experiencing symptoms of psychosis are often unable to think clearly. You should respond to disorganized speech by communicating in an uncomplicated and brief manner, repeating things if necessary. After you say something, you should be patient and allow plenty of time for the person to process the information and respond. If the person is showing a limited range of feelings, you should be aware that this does not mean that the person is not feeling anything. Likewise, you should not assume the person cannot understand what you are saying, even if his or her responses are limited.

Should I Encourage the Person to Seek Professional Help?

You should ask the person if he or she has felt this way before and, if so, what he or she has done in the past that has been helpful. Try to find out what type of assistance the person believes will help him or her. Also, try to determine whether the person has a supportive social network and, if this is the case, encourage him or her to use these supports.

If the person decides to seek professional help, you should make sure that others support him or her both emotionally and practically in accessing services. If the person does seek help, and he or she or you lack confidence in the medical advice received, the person should seek a second opinion from another medical or mental health professional.

What If the Person Does Not Want Help?

The person may refuse to seek help even if that person realizes that he or she is unwell. Confusion and fear about what is happening may lead the person to deny that anything is wrong. In this case, you should encourage the person to talk to someone he or she trusts. It is also possible that a person will refuse to seek help because the person lacks insight that he or she is unwell. The person might actively resist your encouragement to seek help. In either case, your course of action should depend on the type and severity of the person's symptoms.

It is important to recognize that unless a person with psychosis meets the criteria for involuntary commitment (which depends on local, state/provincial, or national laws), others cannot force that person into treatment. Never threaten the person with hospitalization. Instead, remain friendly and open to the possibility that he or she may want your help in the future.

What Should I Do in a Crisis Situation When the Person Has Become Acutely Unwell?

In a crisis situation, you should try to remain as calm as possible. Evaluate the situation by assessing the risks involved (e.g., whether there is any risk that the person will harm himself/herself or others). It is important to assess whether the person is at risk of suicide (see the MHFA Guidelines for Suicidal Behavior, which you can download from www.mhfa.com.au). If the person previously has been in treatment for psychosis and has an **advance directive** or relapse prevention plan, you should follow those instructions. An advance directive is a set of instructions that the person would like followed in the course of a relapse of illness. Try to find out if the person has anyone he or she trusts (e.g., close friends, family) and try to get their help. You should also assess whether it is safe for the person to be alone and, if not, make sure that someone stays with him or her.

It is important to communicate to the person in a way that is clear and to the point and to use short, simple sentences. Speak quietly in a non-threatening tone of voice at a moderate pace. If the person asks you questions, answer them calmly. You should fulfill requests unless they are unsafe or unreasonable. This gives the person the opportunity to feel somewhat in control.

You should be aware that the person might act upon a delusion or hallucination. Remember that your primary task is to de-escalate the situation, so you should not do anything to further upset the person. Try to maintain safety and protect the person, yourself, and others around you from harm. Make sure that you have access to an exit.

You must remain aware that you may not be able to de-escalate the situation, and, if this is the case, you should be prepared to call for assistance. If the person is at risk of harming himself/herself or others, you should make sure that medical or mental health professionals evaluate the person immediately. When assistance arrives, you should convey specific, brief observations about the severity of the person's behavior and symptoms to the emergency responders. You should explain to the person you are helping who any unfamiliar people are, that they are there to help, and how they are going to help. However, if the services you contact dismiss your concerns about the person, you should continue trying to seek help for the individual.

> You must remain aware that you may not be able to de-escalate the situation, and, if this is the case, you should be prepared to call for assistance. If the person is at risk of harming himself/herself or others, you should make sure that medical or mental health professionals evaluate the person immediately.

What If the Person Becomes Aggressive?

People with psychosis are not usually aggressive and are at a much higher risk of harming themselves than others. However, certain symptoms of psychosis (e.g., delusions or hallucinations) can sometimes cause people to become aggressive. You should know how to de-escalate the situation if the person you are trying to help becomes aggressive.

Take any threats or warnings seriously, particularly if the person believes he or she is being persecuted. If you are frightened, seek outside help immediately. You should never put yourself at risk. Similarly, if the person's aggression escalates out of control at any time, you should remove yourself from the situation and call for assistance. When contacting the appropriate mental health service, you should not assume the person is experiencing a specific psychiatric disorder but should instead explain any symptoms and immediate concerns.

If the situation becomes unsafe, it may be necessary to involve the police. To help the police in their response, you should tell them that you believe the person is experiencing a psychotic episode and that you need their help to get medical treatment and to control the person's aggressive behavior. You should tell the police whether or not the person is armed.

How Do I De-escalate the Situation?

- Do not respond to the person in a hostile, disciplinary, or challenging manner.
- Do not threaten him or her as this may increase fear or prompt aggressive behavior.
- Avoid raising your voice or talking too fast.
- Stay calm and avoid nervous behavior (e.g., shuffling your feet, fidgeting, making abrupt movements).
- Do not restrict the person's movement (e.g., if he or she wants to pace up and down the room allow it).
- Remain aware that the symptoms or fear causing the person's aggression might be made worse if you take certain steps (e.g., involve the police).

Key Chapter Points

- Each individual is unique, and it is important to tailor your support to that person's needs.

- You should recognize that the individual may be frightened by his or her thoughts and feelings. Ask the person about what will help him or her to feel safe and in control.

- The person may refuse to seek help even if that person realizes that he or she is unwell.

- You should be aware that the person might act upon a delusion or hallucination. Remember that your primary task is to de-escalate the situation, so you should not do anything to further upset the person.

- If the person is at risk of harming himself/herself or others, you should make sure that mental health professionals evaluate the person immediately.

- If you are frightened, seek outside help immediately. You should never put yourself at risk.

- When contacting the appropriate mental health service, you should not assume the person is experiencing a specific psychiatric illness but should instead explain any symptoms and immediate concerns.

- The role of the first aider is to assist the person until he or she receives appropriate professional help or the crisis resolves.

Glossary

Terms are followed by the number of the chapter in which they first appear.

12-step program (7) – In a 12-step program, an individual follows an ordered list of increasingly challenging tasks that take him or her along the road of recovery from substance abuse. In these programs, someone who has completed the 12 steps often guides a newcomer just beginning the steps through the program. Alcoholics Anonymous is the original 12-step program that forms the basis for similar substance abuse treatment programs.

A

Acetylcholine (6) – Acetylcholine is a neurotransmitter in the brain. Some antipsychotic medicines bind to acetylcholine receptors in the brain, which may lead to some side effects, like dry mouth, constipation, and blurry vision.

Activity groups (7) – Activity groups are a type of group therapy that focuses on experiences and activities. These groups help patients to develop better social skills, confidence, and in some cases, job-related skills.

Acute phase (1) – One of the three phases of psychosis, it is the time during the psychotic episode when symptoms are most disruptive and positive symptoms are present.

Adherence (8) – Adherence means the same thing as compliance with treatment: sticking with the treatment plan and including this treatment plan into one's daily life. It includes taking medicines as prescribed, attending follow-up appointments as scheduled, and completing therapy exercises given at appointments.

Advance directive (16) – An advance directive is a set of instructions that the patient would like followed if a relapse of illness occurs.

Adverse events (6) – Adverse events are similar to side effects in that they are unwanted effects of medicines, but they are much rarer, may happen at any time when taking the medicine, and sometimes may not go away. Also, adverse events are more serious and at times may even be life-threatening. A serious allergic reaction is an example of an adverse event.

Age of onset (1) – The age of onset is the age that psychosis begins. The age of onset of psychosis is usually in late adolescence or early adulthood. For men, the usual age of onset may be slightly earlier (20-30 years) than for women (24–34 years).

Aggressiveness (2) – Most people experiencing psychosis are not dangerous. But some may argue more than normal, destroy property, or make threats towards others. Such behaviors are usually driven by delusions or paranoia.

Anhedonia (2) – Anhedonia is a loss of interest or pleasure. People experiencing this negative symptom may not be able to find pleasure in experiences they used to enjoy. They also may find that they are unable to fully enjoy fun and pleasant things like going to the movies, enjoying a tasty meal, or taking part in hobbies.

Antidepressants (3) – These medicines are used to treat major depression. Like other psychiatric medicines, antidepressants are usually combined with one or more forms of psychotherapy.

Antipsychotics (6) – Antipsychotics are the main types of medicines used to treat psychosis. These medicines are called "antipsychotics" because they fight against ("anti-") psychotic symptoms.

Anxiety (2) – It is common for people experiencing psychosis to be anxious or nervous. One source of anxiety may be delusional thoughts. Anxiety may show up in some people as being tense or jittery, worrying that something bad is going to happen, or appearing uneasy in most situations.

Anxiety medicines (6) – Anxiety medicines are a specific type of psychiatric medicines that may be needed if anxiety symptoms are a problem.

Apathy (2) – Those who have the negative symptom of apathy tend not to care as deeply about what happens in their life. This may include not being upset about negative life events such as losing a job or failing in school.

Assertive community treatment (ACT) (7) – ACT is a psychosocial treatment in which a team of mental health professionals brings treatment opportunities to patients in their own settings. That is, the treatment team comes to the patient (at home), instead of the patient having to come to the treatment team (in a clinic).

Atypical antipsychotics (6) – Atypical antipsychotics is the name used for the newer antipsychotics. They are considered "atypical" for many reasons, but mainly because they cause much less of the movement side effects often seen with the older "conventional" antipsychotic medicines.

Auditory hallucinations (2) – These occur when someone hears voices when there is really no one there. These hallucinations may be voices calling one's name, commenting on one's actions, making harsh comments, or giving commands.

Avolition (9) – Avolition is a negative symptom that is a significant decrease in one's ability to begin and/or follow through with tasks. People with avolition may be unable to finish tasks or complete them on time.

B

Bipolar disorder (3) – A mental health professional gives a diagnosis of bipolar disorder when someone has had one or more episodes of mania. Episodes of major depression may happen between the episodes of mania.

Bizarre behaviors (2) – People with psychosis may do things that do not make any sense and look like random, odd behaviors.

Blunted affect (2) – People with blunted affect show less outward emotion than normal. This is observed as decreased facial expression, less body language, and a bland tone of voice. This negative symptom is also known as decreased expression of emotion.

Brief, intermittent hallucinations (9) – Examples of brief, intermittent hallucinations include briefly hearing a name called out loud that no one else can hear or seeing an object or person for a few seconds that no one else can see. These hallucinations happen only occasionally. They may be prodromal symptoms before the first episode of psychosis or early warning signs before a relapse of psychosis.

Brief psychotic disorder (3) – People with this disorder have one or more positive symptoms, but these symptoms last only from one day to one month.

C

Candidate genes (4) – Candidate genes are genes that might increase one's risk for a disorder like psychosis. But further research is needed.

Case management (14) – Case management is a treatment service in which one person is in charge of checking in with the patient on a regular basis and making sure that he or she has all the services needed. It's an important part of many programs designed especially for people with psychosis.

Catatonia (2) – Catatonia is a severe change from normal body movements that happens without a clear reason. Although catatonia is rare, it sometimes occurs with psychosis. People who experience catatonia may have difficulty moving, appearing frozen, stiff, and motionless.

Civil commitment (5) – In civil commitment, the patient has symptoms that require hospitalization, but he or she does not agree to sign into the hospital. A psychiatrist or psychologist can keep the patient in the hospital, depending on local, state/provincial, or national laws. This is also called involuntary inpatient treatment, involuntary hospitalization, or compulsory treatment.

Cognitive abilities (2) – Cognitive abilities are the abilities to understand, process, and recall information. Cognitive abilities include attention, learning, memory, and planning.

Cognitive-behavioral therapy (CBT) (7) – CBT is a type of therapy sometimes used for people experiencing an episode of psychosis that targets the specific thoughts and beliefs that an individual has that make symptoms worse.

Cognitive dysfunction (2) – This term refers to symptoms that cause problems with understanding, processing, and recalling information. Although people with psychosis typically have a relatively normal intelligence or IQ (intelligence quotient), they may have some problems with other cognitive abilities.

Cognitive remediation (7) – This type of individual therapy or counseling may use games and exercises. Cognitive remediation may be helpful in improving cognitive dysfunction, including difficulties in attention, learning, memory, and planning.

Cognitive tasks (5) – Cognitive tasks include things such as remembering items or putting items into categories. Psychiatrists and psychologists use these tests to assess a patient's cognitive abilities and whether or not cognitive dysfunction may be present. When used in a specialized imaging study, doctors can determine how different parts of the brain are functioning based on blood flow to those areas.

Cognitive tests (2) – A group of tests doctors use to assess for cognitive dysfunction. They are also known as neurocognitive tests, neuropsychological tests, or psychological tests.

Collateral information (5) – Collateral information is additional information gathered by mental health professionals that may confirm the patient's history or provide another perspective on recent problems. Mental health professionals want this information to get several views on what has been going on.

Comorbidity (7) – Comorbidity, co-occurring disorders, or dual diagnosis all mean that two illnesses happen at the same time. In the context of psychosis, these terms often mean that psychosis occurs at the same time as a substance abuse problem.

Compliance (8) – Compliance refers to patients sticking with their treatment plan and including this treatment plan into their daily life. Compliance is the same as adherence.

Compliance therapy (7) – A type of individual therapy or counseling that aims to increase a patient's abilities to regularly take medicine and attend follow-up appointments.

Compulsory treatment (5) – In compulsory treatment, the patient has symptoms that require hospitalization, but he or she does not agree to sign into the hospital. A psychiatrist or psychologist can keep the patient in the hospital, depending on local, state/provincial, or national laws. This is also called involuntary inpatient treatment, involuntary hospitalization, or civil commitment.

Computerized axial tomography (CAT) scan (5) – A CAT scan is commonly used as part of the initial evaluation. It is similar to a very detailed x-ray of the brain. It is also known as a computerized tomography (CT) scan.

Consumer (11) – In the recovery movement, patients are often called consumers. This means that they choose which services they will use and how they will use the available services. Consumers themselves decide on their personal goals for treatment and recovery instead of mental health professionals deciding for them.

Conventional antipsychotics (6) – This name is used for the older types of antipsychotics. The newer antipsychotics are often referred to as atypical antipsychotics.

Co-occurring disorders (7) – Co-occurring disorders, comorbidity, or dual diagnosis all mean that two illnesses happen at the same time. In the context of psychosis, these terms often mean that psychosis occurs at the same time as a substance abuse problem.

Coping (13) – Coping means facing and dealing with responsibilities, problems, or difficulties in a successful and calm manner.

Critical period (1) – Some researchers think of the first five years during and after a first episode of psychosis as a critical period. That is, the early phase of psychosis is very important because it is during this time that long-term outcome may be most improved by treatment. This is also a critical period because psychological and social skills are developing and mental health professionals want to minimize the damage to psychological and social skills that psychosis can cause.

D

Day/night reversal (9) – Unlike insomnia or hypersomnia, people with day/night reversal get the same amount of sleep as usual but stay awake at night and sleep during the day. People with psychosis sometimes have this sleep pattern.

Day treatment programs (7) – Day treatment programs are outpatient treatment facilities that provide daytime (but not overnight) treatment to individuals diagnosed with psychosis and other mental illnesses. Both day treatment and partial hospitalization provide a more intensive form of treatment than usual outpatient clinic appointments without requiring overnight hospital stays.

Decreased expression of emotion (9) – Decreased expression of emotion, also called blunted affect, is a negative symptom in which the "usual" expression of emotion decreases or is lessened.

Delirium (3) – Delirium is a state of confusion that develops rapidly, over the course of hours or days. It is usually due to a medical condition, taking a drug of abuse, or withdrawing from certain drugs. Unlike psychosis, delirium often causes disorientation.

Delusional disorder (3) – Delusional disorder is similar to schizophrenia, except the main symptom is a single delusion. It is quite rare, but when it does happen, it tends to be somewhat less severe than schizophrenia.

Delusion of control (2) – A type of delusion in which people believe that some other person or an outside force controls their thoughts, feelings, or actions.

Delusions (2) – Delusions are fixed, false beliefs. Delusions are a form of so-called "positive" symptoms of schizophrenia and related psychotic disorders.

Dementia (3) – Dementia causes confusion and disorientation, developing slowly over the course of months or years. Dementia usually occurs in older people, typically after the age of 65 years, and often after the age of 80 years. The most common form of dementia is Alzheimer's disease.

Depressed mood (2) – People with depressed mood, also simply called depression, feel down, unhappy, or empty.

Depression (2) – Depression is another common term for depressed mood. It is also a common term for a psychiatric illness, major depression.

Derailment (2) – In this form of disorganized thinking, one idea connects to the next, but the thoughts become confusing because they go off on a tangent and end on a different subject.

Deterioration in role functioning (9) – A deterioration in role functioning happens when people become less able to carry out daily activities due to an illness. These activities can include work, family responsibilities, household chores, personal hygiene, recreation, and socializing.

Diagnosis (2) – A diagnosis (plural: diagnoses) is the specific medical word(s) given to an illness or syndrome by health-care providers.

Diagnostic and Statistical Manual of Mental Disorders (DSM) (3) – This book is published by the American Psychiatric Association and used by mental health professionals in making a psychiatric diagnosis. Another classification of mental illnesses is the International Classification of Diseases.

Diathesis-stress model (1) – This model about the development of psychosis suggests that psychosis happens because of the relationship between one's genes and the environment one lives in. The diathesis refers to one's genetic risk, and the stress refers to the external risk factors that are not genetic.

Differential diagnosis (3) – Doctors create this list of the most likely reasons for a health problem, in this case, psychosis. The list helps doctors decide on the most likely diagnosis.

Difficulties with abstract thinking (2) – Some people with psychosis may not be able to understand complex concepts or solve problems that require them to think through several steps. Also, they may find it difficult to understand abstract meanings, as in proverbs or sayings.

Difficulties with planning (2) – The cognitive changes experienced with psychosis may make it hard to plan. A person may have trouble focusing on future events in a logical way. He or she may also not have the ability to correctly judge different plans of action. In addition, they may become uncertain and have difficulty committing to one plan and following through with it.

Disorganization (2) – The normal flow of thinking and speaking can become out of order, confusing, and jumbled. Disorganized thinking is a major category of symptoms of psychosis.

Disorganized behavior (2) – Disorganized behavior appears as an inability to follow through with plans or as an odd appearance or behavior. For example, the patient may have shoes on the wrong feet or wear clothes inside out. As another example, people with disorganized behavior may dress inappropriately for the weather, often wearing several layers of clothing, even in warm temperatures.

Disorientation (3) – Not knowing the time, place, or situation. This form of confusion can be seen in people with delirium and dementia.

Dopamine (4) – Dopamine is a neurotransmitter, a natural chemical in the brain that allows certain neurons to communicate with one another. Psychosis may be caused by a dysfunction in some dopamine pathways.

Drug-induced psychosis (1) – Drug-induced psychosis may happen when a person is using drugs like marijuana, cocaine, LSD, PCP, or methamphetamine.

Dual-diagnosis (7) – Patients with a dual-diagnosis have a diagnosis of both a psychotic disorder and a substance use disorder. Other terms sometimes used for dual-diagnosis are comorbidity or co-occurring disorders, which also mean that two illnesses happen at the same time, in this case a psychotic disorder and an addiction.

Dual-diagnosis program (7) – A dual-diagnosis program is a treatment, often in an inpatient or residential setting (meaning that the patient lives there for several weeks or months), that focuses on helping individuals who not only have a diagnosed mental illness but also have a substance abuse problem. These programs treat both problems.

Dysphoria (9) – Dysphoria is another word for sadness.

E

Early warning signs (9) – Changes in thoughts, feelings, and behaviors that happen a few days or weeks before an episode of psychosis may be early warning signs. It is important for patients and their families to be familiar with their specific early warning signs because recognizing these signs may help in preventing a relapse.

Electroencephalogram (EEG) (5) – An EEG records the electrical activity in the brain. To do the EEG, the clinician will attach a number of small electrodes and wires to the person's scalp. The EEG is painless and is commonly used to make sure that seizures are not happening.

Emotional withdrawal (2) – People with emotional withdrawal lack emotional closeness to others. They do not feel like they belong or connect with others, even when spending time with other people. Emotional withdrawal is a so-called "negative" symptom of schizophrenia and related psychotic disorders.

Evaluation (5) – A thorough evaluation is the first step for mental health professionals to help people experiencing a first psychotic episode. The main reason for evaluation is to better understand what people with psychosis are experiencing. In an evaluation, the mental health professional will interview and observe the person, gather records that may be helpful, contact others who know the patient to get their perspectives, and do a number of medical and psychological exams.

Extrapyramidal side effects (EPS) (6) – EPS are a number of movement side effects, which can be quite common when taking conventional antipsychotics. They are much less likely to occur when taking the newer atypical antipsychotic medicines.

F

Family interventions (7) – Family interventions help families to cope with stress, improve their social supports, and reduce the effects of stigma. Such interventions view each member of the family as having an important role or purpose. Family interventions include family psychoeducation and family therapy.

Family psychoeducation (7) – Family psychoeducation is a type of family intervention that educates family members about early psychosis and the types of experiences that they can expect when a loved one has psychosis. It may take place within a single family or within multi-family groups.

Family therapy (7) – Family therapy, a form of family intervention, focuses not only on educating the family about psychosis (as in family psychoeducation), but also on improving communication and problem-solving skills.

Fasting glucose and lipids (6) – Because of the possibility of some side effects, doctors prescribing atypical antipsychotics closely monitor the patient's weight and periodically check certain labs, like fasting glucose (sugar) and lipids. This requires drawing a sample of blood to be sent to the lab.

First-episode psychosis (1) – First-episode psychosis is the period of time when a person first begins to experience psychosis.

Flat affect (2) – Flat affect is an extreme lessening of outward emotion (even more severe than blunted affect). People show this negative symptom of schizophrenia and related psychotic disorders by an almost complete absence of facial expression and body language and a very bland tone of voice.

Functional magnetic resonance imaging (fMRI) (5) – This specialized type of MRI, used for research to measure blood flow in the brain, helps to determine how the brain is functioning.

G

Generic name (6) – A generic name is one of two names of a medicine. For example, acetaminophen is the generic name for Tylenol.

Genes (4) – Genes are segments of DNA that pass along the "blueprints" of how the body's cells are to make proteins.

Glutamate (4) – Glutamate is a neurotransmitter in the brain. People with psychosis may have a dysfunction in glutamate pathways.

Grandiose delusion (2) – The false belief that one has really high social status, is famous, has large amounts of money, or has special powers.

Group therapy (7) – Group therapy is a psychosocial treatment in which one or two mental health professionals lead a group of patients in a discussion or a planned activity. It allows patients to learn not only from the therapist, but also from the interactions between the therapist and other patients, and between other patients and themselves.

H

Hallucinations (2) – A hallucination is experiencing something that is not really there, like hearing a voice that is not really there (an auditory hallucination) or seeing something that is not really there (a visual hallucination). Hallucinations are a type of the so-called "positive" symptoms of schizophrenia and related psychotic disorders.

Heritable (4) – Heritable means that an illness is partly caused by genes. Many illnesses that those psychosis, like schizophrenia, are heritable, or partly caused by genes, even though they may not appear to run in families.

Histamine (6) – Histamine is a neurotransmitter in the brain. Some antipsychotics may bind to histamine receptors in the brain, which may lead to side effects like sleepiness.

History (5) – Doctors do a history and a physical exam as part of the evaluation of a medical condition like psychosis. The history includes a large amount of information, taken from the interview, about what has been going on in the past and recently.

Hostility (2) – Most people experiencing psychosis are not dangerous. But some argue more than normal, destroy property, or make threats towards others. Such behaviors are usually driven by paranoia, delusions, or other symptoms.

Hypersomnia (9) – Hypersomnia means sleeping more than usual. It is the opposite of insomnia.

I

Ideas of reference (2) – In this positive symptom of psychosis, patients believe that people are talking about them or are referring to them when they are really not.

Imaging studies (5) – Imaging studies allow radiologists and mental health professionals to look at the brain to determine if there are any abnormal findings, such as brain tumors or infections. Such imaging studies are also called neuroimaging.

Impaired information processing (2) – People experiencing this form of cognitive dysfunction have difficulty sorting out information and discovering meaning in things that they observe. It may appear that things do not "sink in" or that complex things seem more difficult for them to understand than before.

Impaired insight (2) – People experiencing psychotic symptoms often are not fully aware of their behavior or the condition of their mind. Because their unusual experiences may be very real to them, they do not realize that their thoughts and behaviors are a change from their normal self.

Inappropriate affect (2) – A symptom in which one repeatedly smiles or laughs out of context. This symptom is often seen in bipolar disorder or in schizophrenia—disorganized type.

Inpatient (5) – Inpatient treatment settings are usually in hospitals, and patients usually stay overnight for several days. The amount of time spent depends on how serious the individual's symptoms are.

Insomnia (9) – Insomnia is a difficulty in sleeping, such as taking more than 30 minutes to fall asleep or waking up in the middle of the night and not being able to go back to sleep. It can also be waking up more than 30 minutes earlier in the morning than normal.

Integrated treatment programs (7) – Mental health professionals in these programs focus on both the treatment of psychosis and substance abuse at the same time in the same setting.

International Classification of Diseases (ICD) (3) – This classification used by mental health professionals provides specific definitions of psychiatric disorders and is produced by the World Health Organization. Another classification of mental illnesses is the Diagnostic and Statistical Manual of Mental Disorders (DSM), produced by the American Psychiatric Association.

Interview (5) – An interview with the patient by a psychiatrist or psychologist is the first step in an evaluation. This interview helps the mental health professional to understand the difficulties the patient has been experiencing.

Involuntary hospitalization (5) – The patient enters the hospital even if he or she does not recognize the need for treatment. This is also called involuntary inpatient treatment, civil commitment, or compulsory treatment.

Involuntary inpatient treatment (5) – In involuntary inpatient treatment, the patient has symptoms that require hospitalization, but he or she does not agree to sign in to the hospital. A psychiatrist or psychologist may keep the patient in the hospital, depending on local, state/provincial, or national laws. This is also called involuntary hospitalization, civil commitment, or compulsory treatment.

L

Labile affect (2) – This occurs when a person's mood quickly changes between happy and sad, such as laughing that quickly switches to crying. It is commonly seen during an episode of mania in bipolar disorder, but may also be present in schizophrenia and related psychotic disorders.

Language problems (2) – People with psychosis may have trouble writing or speaking. Language problems also may include using words incorrectly, using new words that do not really have a true meaning, or using words because of what they sound like instead of what they mean.

Life events (13) – Life events are one kind of stressor and include things such as becoming ill, experiencing the death of a loved one, going through a divorce, getting married, having a baby, getting a new job, or moving. Some life events are more stressful than others.

Loosening of association (2) – In this form of disorganized thinking, one idea does not match the next. Ideas shift from one subject to another in a completely unrelated way. The thinking process is "loose" instead of being tightly ordered and reasonable.

Low drive, energy, or motivation (2) – Those experiencing this negative symptom may have lost the desire to finish school, get a job, or engage in social activities.

Lumbar puncture (5) – This medical procedure is performed by doctors to rule out an infection in the brain by examining cerebrospinal fluid. It is also known as a spinal tap.

M

Magical thinking (9) – Magical thinking can involve such things as wondering about the ability to read others' minds or believing in superstition too much. Magical thinking may be a mild form of a positive symptom like delusions and may be a prodromal symptom or an early warning sign of a relapse of psychosis.

Magnetic resonance imaging (MRI) (5) – An imaging study, or form of neuroimaging, that allows mental health professionals to see any abnormalities, such as tumors, swelling inside the brain, or small areas of disease that might cause psychotic symptoms. The MRI uses magnetic waves instead of X-ray radiation.

Major depression (3) – Major depression, also called major depressive disorder or clinical depression, is when one has been feeling depressed and has a number of depressive symptoms for at least two weeks. A depressive episode may last weeks, months, or even years.

Mania (2) – Mania is an episode of abnormally excited mood, such as periods in which the person feels abnormally good, high, or excited. People who have a manic episode often receive a diagnosis of bipolar disorder.

Medical record (5) – The medical record documents the evaluation and treatments that are prescribed. It also helps mental health professionals communicate with one another about the patient's progress. The medical record is confidential, based on local, state/provincial, or national laws.

Mental illness (1) – A mental illness is a health condition that affects a person's thoughts, feelings, and behaviors. Like physical illnesses, mental illnesses are treatable.

Mental status exam (5) – A mental status exam is part of the interview done by a mental health professional during an evaluation. The mental status exam includes an assessment of several aspects of mental functioning, including appearance, attitude, behavior, speech, mood, affect, thought process, thought content, insight, judgment, impulse control, and cognition.

Metabolic side effects (6) – Antipsychotic medicines can sometimes cause metabolic side effects, which include elevations in blood sugar and cholesterol levels. Doctors monitor for these side effects because they can have negative effects on long-term health.

Mobile crisis teams (14) – Mobile teams usually include several people who go to talk with someone who may have psychosis or another mental illness or crisis. They may go to the person's school, home, or wherever else he or she may be. Mobile teams sometimes also work closely with hotlines or police departments.

Mood stabilizers (3) – These medicines are used to treat bipolar disorder in combination with certain types of psychotherapy. They may also be useful if irritability, impulsiveness, hostility, or unstable moods are present even if bipolar disorder is not diagnosed.

Mood symptoms (2) – Changes in one's moods or feelings may come before or appear with psychosis. Some people may experience a depressed mood, or depression. Others may experience the syndrome of mania.

Motivational enhancement therapy (10) – Motivational enhancement therapy is a treatment to help patients quit smoking by increasing their desire or motivation to quit. It can also be used to increase motivation in other areas, like adherence with treatment.

Movement symptoms (2) – Movement symptoms, a change from normal body movements that happens without a clear reason, can sometimes occur during a psychotic episode.

Multi-family groups (7) – In this form of family psychoeducation, family members from several different families that are going through the same thing are present. This is helpful because family members can talk to other families who also have a loved one experiencing a psychotic disorder. The patient may or may not be present when family psychoeducation takes place in multi-family groups.

N

Negative symptoms (2) – Negative symptoms are things that people should normally do or think that are now missing. These symptoms have subtracted or removed something from their experience. Negative symptoms are one of the major types of signs and symptoms of psychotic disorders.

Neurodevelopmental model (1) – The neurodevelopmental model posits that psychosis is the result of minor injuries to or abnormalities in the brain during its growth and development.

Neuroimaging (5) – Neuroimaging allow radiologists and mental health professionals to look at the brain to determine if there are any abnormal findings, such as brain tumors or infections. These medical procedures are also called imaging studies.

Neurons (4) – Neurons are cells in the brain.

Neurotransmitters (4) – The substances needed for communication between neurons in the brain.

Nicotine replacement therapy (10) – Nicotine replacement therapy can be very helpful for someone trying to stop smoking. Types of nicotine replacement include a gum, patch, or inhaler. These nondangerous substitutions make it easier to quit smoking.

Nonadherent (8) – Patients are nonadherent when they do not stick with their treatment plan or try to include this plan into their daily life. The term *noncompliant* means the same thing.

Noninvasive (5) – Medical tests that are noninvasive do not involve any needles, incisions, or entry into the body.

Norepinephrine (6) – Norepinephrine is a neurotransmitter in the brain. Some antipsychotics may bind to norepinephrine receptors, and this may cause certain side effects, like low blood pressure.

O

Observation (5) – During an evaluation, in addition to completing a thorough interview, the mental health professional observes the patient's behavior. Such observations include watching the patient's facial expression, movements, and body language.

Ongoing stressors (13) – Ongoing stressors are a part of everyone's life. Some of these include unwanted or unpleasant household chores, frequent or repeated arguments or conflicts, financial problems, constant criticism, or a chronic illness in a loved one.

Outpatient (5) – Patients in an outpatient setting visit the treatment facility for an appointment, but then return home.

Outpatient commitment (5) – A court order may be used to ensure that the patient stays in outpatient treatment. If he or she fails to continue outpatient treatment, then hospitalization may be necessary.

Outpatient commitment is also called involuntary community treatment.

Overvalued ideas (9) – An overvalued idea is a mild form of a positive symptom in which too much emphasis is placed on an idea. Overvalued ideas can involve religious, philosophical, or any other type of idea that one is overly concerned with. Sometimes overvalued ideas may be prodromal symptoms or may be an early warning signs that occurs before a relapse of psychosis.

P

Paranoia (2) – People with this positive symptom of psychosis feel that they cannot trust others. They may have an unexplained feeling that those around them are trying to cause problems in their life.

Paranoid delusion (2) – A paranoid delusion is a fixed, false belief that one is being plotted against or followed.

Paranoid schizophrenia (3) – Paranoid schizophrenia (also called schizophrenia—paranoid type) means that the person's symptoms mainly consist of delusions and/or auditory hallucinations. This is probably the most common form of schizophrenia.

Partial hospitalization (7) – Partial hospitalization programs are outpatient treatment programs that provide daytime (but not overnight) treatment to individuals diagnosed with psychosis and other mental illnesses. Partial hospitalization, like day treatment, provides a more intensive form of treatment than usual outpatient clinic appointments without requiring overnight hospital stays.

Perceptual abnormality (9) – A perceptual abnormality is the experience of one of the five senses (hearing, seeing, feeling, tasting, or smelling) changing such that the person wonders if the mind might be playing tricks on him or her. A perceptual abnormality is a mild form of a hallucination that may be a prodromal symptom or an early warning sign of a relapse of psychosis.

Phase-specific care (14) – Researchers now believe that providing phase-specific care is best for patients with a first episode of psychosis. This means that the treatment plan for each individual patient is tailored to his or her own needs, depending on the kinds of symptoms present, how severe the symptoms are, and the types of other problems going on in the patient's life.

Poor attention and concentration (2) – People experiencing psychosis often display limited attention and concentration. They may have a hard time keeping their mind on one idea. They also may find tasks that require them to focus their attention very tiring. Poor attention and concentration is a form of cognitive dysfunction.

Poor attention to grooming and hygiene (2) – This can include not bathing or brushing one's teeth, wearing dirty clothes, not combing one's hair, etc. This self-neglect can be a negative symptom of psychotic disorders.

Poor memory (2) – People with psychosis may have difficulty remembering past events. Some also may have trouble learning and remembering new things. Poor memory is a form of cognitive dysfunction that may be present with psychosis.

Positive symptoms (2) – Positive symptoms of schizophrenia and related psychotic disorders are experiences that people should not normally have. In other words, these symptoms have added something to their experience. Positive symptoms include hallucinations, delusions, and paranoia.

Positron emission tomography (PET) scan (5) – This type of research imaging study used to measure blood flow in the brain helps to determine how the brain is functioning.

Postpartum psychosis (3) – Mental health professionals give a diagnosis of postpartum psychosis when a woman begins having psychotic symptoms anytime within the first three months after giving birth. The symptoms usually begin within the first month after the child's birth and usually come on fairly suddenly.

Poverty of content of speech (2) – A negative symptom in which the thought patterns may become unclear, meaningless, or empty.

Primary psychotic disorders (3) – This group of psychotic disorders primarily cause psychosis, rather than depression, anxiety, or another type of syndrome.

Prodromal phase (1) – One of the three phases of psychosis. It is the time before a psychotic episode when early symptoms first begin.

Prodromal symptoms (2) – These are changes in thoughts, feelings, or behaviors that happen before an episode of psychosis begins.

Prolactin (6) – Prolactin is a hormone secreted by the pituitary gland in the brain. When taking conventional antipsychotics, and some atypical antipsychotics, the prolactin level in the blood may rise. This may cause some side effects.

Pruning (4) – Synaptic pruning produces more efficient connections between neurons in the brain by reducing the number of "weak" connections between neurons. This is a normal process of brain development that may be particularly important in childhood and adolescence.

Psychiatrist (5) – A psychiatrist is a doctor who has received training in medicine. Psychiatrists evaluate and treat people with mental illnesses and often prescribe medicines as part of the treatment.

Psychoeducation (15) – A type of education that focuses on the topic of mental illnesses with the goal of helping individuals with a mental illness, and their family members, to better understand the illness.

Psychoeducational groups (7) – Psychoeducational groups are a type of group therapy that teach patients about their illness in a clear, structured way, similar to a small classroom. In psychoeducational groups, patients learn from mental health professionals about symptoms, treatments, early warning signs, and other topics relevant to psychosis.

Psychologist (5) – A psychologist is a doctor who has received training in psychology. Although psychologists are usually not licensed to prescribe medicines, they have other skills, such as performing formal psychological testing.

Psychosis (1) – Psychosis refers to a mental state of being out of touch with reality. It is a medical condition that occurs due to a dysfunction in the brain. People with psychosis have difficulty separating false personal experiences from reality. That is, they may have symptoms like hallucinations or delusions.

Psychosis continuum (1) – The psychosis continuum refers to the different levels of psychotic experiences. This simply means that there is a range of severity across the different types of experiences of psychosis. This range is from normal experiences similar to psychosis to the full syndrome of psychosis that greatly interferes with one's life.

Psychosis-prone (1) – People are said to be psychosis-prone when they are particularly at risk for psychosis based on their genes or due to exposure to environmental factors that may have occurred in early life.

Psychosis related to a medical problem (1) – People with a physical illness, such as meningitis, seizures, or brain tumors, may experience psychosis related to the medical problem.

Psychosocial development (7) – Normal development of psychological and social skills begins in childhood but continues throughout adolescence and early adulthood, which is an extremely important time when most people develop social skills and build relationships.

Psychosocial problems (7) – Psychosocial problems refer to difficulties at school, at work, in relationships, or in recreation and leisure activities. Psychosocial problems may come about when someone does not have the skills needed to successfully interact with his or her social environment. Psychosis often causes major psychosocial problems.

Psychosocial rehabilitation (7) – Mental health professionals sometimes use the term psychosocial rehabilitation to describe many psychosocial treatments. This means that treatment increases psychosocial skills to the best possible level of functioning.

Psychosocial treatments (7) – These are treatments that focus on helping patients with psychosocial problems (like difficulties with school, work, relationships, and recreation/leisure activities).

Psychotic (1) – The word psychotic describes someone who is experiencing the condition of psychosis, having either hallucinations or delusions.

Psychotic disorder (1) – A psychotic disorder is a mental illness that brings about psychosis that interferes with life. Some people diagnosed with a psychotic disorder will have repeated episodes with periods of normal functioning in between, while others may experience only one episode in their lifetime.

Psychotic disorder not otherwise specified (psychotic disorder NOS) (3) – People diagnosed with psychotic disorder NOS have psychotic symptoms but the mental health professional does not have enough information to make a more specific diagnosis. It is often used as a preliminary diagnosis by mental health professionals before deciding on a final diagnosis.

Psychotic episode (1) – A psychotic episode is a period of time during which someone has psychotic symptoms. The length of a psychotic episode differs from person to person.

Public stigma (12) – Others' negative beliefs about mental illnesses that lead to discrimination.

R

Rapport (7) – Good rapport is a good working relationship with one's therapist or mental health professional.

Reality testing (7) – Reality testing refers to one's ability to decide between what is real and what is not real. Because psychosis refers to a mental state of being out of touch with reality, someone who is psychotic has an impairment in reality testing (e.g., hearing voices or having false beliefs).

Receptors (6) – Receptors are proteins on the surface of cells, such as nerve cells or neurons. Medicines bind to receptors once they are in the brain.

Recovery (8) – The goal of the recovery process is to empower individuals to achieve their fullest potential in life. The recovery philosophy embraces the belief that one can achieve identified and declared life goals when given freedom and support, as well as necessary information, education, and skills sets. Recovery is a broader goal of treatment than just remission of symptoms.

Recovery model (3) – The recovery model aims to empower the patient to achieve his or her own goals by actively participating in treatment decisions.

Recovery phase (1) – One of the three phases of psychosis, it is the time after the psychotic episode when symptoms of psychosis lessen or sometimes go away completely with treatment. The recovery phase is usually considered to be roughly the first 6–18 months of treatment.

Referral (7) – A referral is when a health care professional recommends that a patient goes to a particular type of treatment.

Relapse (2) – A relapse is when psychotic symptoms reappear.

Relapse prevention (9) – Relapse prevention is the goal of preventing psychotic symptoms from coming back by remaining in treatment and watching for early warning signs.

Religious delusion (2) – A fixed, false belief in which one believes that he or she has religious powers or is a biblical or religious figure.

Remission (6) – Remission from psychosis means the major symptoms, usually positive symptoms like hallucinations and delusions, are no longer active. Remission focuses on symptoms, whereas recovery focuses on the patient's own life goals.

Risk factors (4) – A risk factor is any event, exposure, or entity that occurs before the illness and that research has shown plays a role in causing the illness. For example, cigarette smoking is a well-known risk factor for lung cancer. Research has identified a number of risk factors for psychosis.

Risk genes (4) – Risk genes are genes that each play a small role in a person's likelihood of developing psychosis.

S

Schizoaffective disorder (3) – People diagnosed with schizoaffective disorder have a combination of psychotic symptoms as well as serious mood symptoms. There are two types: bipolar type and depressive type.

Schizoaffective disorder—bipolar type (3) – People diagnosed with this type of schizoaffective disorder have symptoms of schizophrenia but also have symptoms of mania.

Schizoaffective disorder—depressive type (3) – People diagnosed with this type of schizoaffective disorder have symptoms of schizophrenia but also have symptoms of depression.

Schizophrenia (3) – People with schizophrenia have a combination of psychotic symptoms (two or more of the following: delusions, hallucinations, disorganized speech, disorganized or catatonic behavior, and negative symptoms), and the illness lasts for at least six months.

Schizophrenia—catatonic type (3) – In schizophrenia—catatonic type, the individual has catatonia. This type of schizophrenia is relatively rare.

Schizophrenia—disorganized type (3) – The diagnosis of schizophrenia—disorganized type means that the person has disorganized speech, disorganized behavior, and flat or inappropriate affect.

Schizophrenia—paranoid type (3) – Schizophrenia—paranoid type (also called paranoid schizophrenia) means that the person's symptoms mainly consist of delusions and/or auditory hallucinations. This is probably the most common form of schizophrenia.

Schizophrenia—residual type (3) – People diagnosed with schizophrenia—residual type have clearly had a psychotic episode diagnosable as schizophrenia in the past, but currently do not have any positive symptoms (like hallucinations or delusions). However, milder forms of symptoms and prominent negative symptoms are still present.

Schizophrenia—undifferentiated type (3) – A person is diagnosed with schizophrenia—undifferentiated type when the mental health professional is sure that the individual has schizophrenia, but the symptoms do not fit into any of three other types (paranoid type, disorganized type, or catatonic type).

Schizophreniform disorder (3) – People diagnosed with this disorder have a combination of psychotic symptoms (two or more of the following: delusions, hallucinations, disorganized speech, disorganized or catatonic behavior, and negative symptoms) that last at least one month but do not continue for more than six months.

Schizotypal personality disorder (3) – Most mental health professionals think of schizotypal personality disorder as a mild form of schizophrenia that never leads to the full syndrome of psychosis. The person may seem odd and eccentric, but not psychotic.

Schizotypal personality features (1) – People who experience mild, ongoing difficulties from psychotic-like symptoms, but can still function well enough to work and maintain relationships, may have schizotypal personality features.

Self stigma (12) – Self stigma is when someone with a mental illness holds negative attitudes about mental illnesses.

Serotonin (6) – Serotonin is a natural chemical in the brain, a neurotransmitter, that plays a role in the mental functions affected by psychosis, anxiety, and depression.

Severity (1) – Severity refers to the levels of seriousness of things such as symptoms and experiences of psychosis.

Shared psychotic disorder (3) – In this very rare diagnosis, a person develops a delusion while in a close relationship with another person who already has a similar established delusion, as in delusional disorder.

Side effects (6) – Side effects are unwanted effects of medicines.

Signs (2) – Signs are like symptoms but a doctor sees them through an interview, an examination, or a test, instead of the patient experiencing and expressing them. The patient may not even know that they have signs of an illness.

Single photon emission computed tomography (SPECT) scan (5) – This type of research imaging study is used to measure blood flow in the brain, helping to determine how the brain is functioning.

Sleep medicines (6) – Sleep medicines are sometimes used to treat insomnia. They may be needed if people with psychosis have difficulty sleeping.

Slow movements (2) – People showing slow movements may walk and move much more slowly than normal. This may be a negative symptom of psychotic disorders.

Slow or empty thinking and speech (2) – This negative symptom may cause the patient to have trouble with conversation. It may seem like the person is unable to keep up with the conversation. There may also be a long period between asking someone a question and his or her response to it.

Smoking cessation (10) – The process of quitting smoking.

Smoking cessation medicines (10) – Medicines are available to make quitting smoking easier. These include bupropion (Wellbutrin, Zyban) and varenicline (Chantix).

Social isolation (2) – Those experiencing this negative symptom may become unconcerned with relationships that had been close and important to them. They usually have difficulty forming new relationships and may instead spend their time alone.

Social skills (7) – Social skills are the daily skills that allow us to successfully interact with one another and have rewarding relationships. Good social skills allow us to have close, supportive relationships with others. Developing psychotic symptoms often disrupts the normal process of social development and interferes with the maturation of social skills.

Social skills training (7) – Social skills training is a psychosocial treatment that helps patients to regain their prior level of social skills or to resume development of social skills interrupted by psychosis. It focuses on problem solving and works to increase social adjustment of patients with psychosis, without necessarily focusing on symptoms alone.

Social withdrawal (9) – People who have this early warning sign or negative symptom are generally not interested in having social contact with others and are less likely to become involved socially.

Somatic delusion (2) – The fixed, false belief that something is wrong with one's body.

Spinal tap (5) – This medical procedure is performed by doctors to rule out an infection in the brain by examining cerebrospinal fluid. It is also known as a lumbar puncture.

Stereotypes (12) – Negative ideas about a person, related to stigma in society.

Stigma (12) – A society's stereotypes, misbeliefs, and discrimination towards certain groups of people, such as those with a mental illness.

Stress (13) – The word stress describes a feeling of strain, pressure, or tension.

Stressful life events (4) – Various stressful life events may be risk factors for schizophrenia or may worsen the symptoms of psychosis. Such difficulties may include child abuse, discrimination, poverty, and the sense of "social defeat" that these problems may lead to.

Stress-induced psychosis (1) – People who experience a great deal of physical stress from lack of sleep, hunger, or torture may experience stress-induced psychosis.

Stressors (13) – Stressors are events that cause stress. In general, there are two types of stressors, life events and ongoing stressors.

Substance use disorder (10) – This diagnosis is given when excessive use of substances interferes with an individual's ability to perform on the job, disrupts his or her relationships, or results in legal problems. Abused substances can include alcohol or drugs like marijuana or cocaine.

Supported education (7) – This approach that is being considered by some researchers would support patients with first-episode psychosis in late adolescence or early adulthood to complete their education.

Supported employment (7) – This type of vocational rehabilitation helps individuals with psychosis find and keep a job. Supported employment programs allow people with serious mental illnesses to work either part-time or full-time, while keeping job stress at a minimum.

Supportive housing (7) – This type of psychosocial treatment provides a safe, supportive place to live for patients with serious mental illnesses.

Supportive psychotherapy (7) – A type of individual therapy or counseling that supports the patient's best coping skills.

Suicidal thoughts (2) – Such thoughts include wishing to be dead or thinking or planning to commit suicide.

Suspiciousness (2) – Suspiciousness is a feeling that one cannot trust others or the unexplained feeling that others are trying to cause problems in one's life.

Symptom (2) – A symptom is an obvious change from a person's normal health that indicates that an illness or disease may be present. Symptoms differ from signs in that symptoms are experienced by the person himself or herself.

Syndrome (2) – A combination of both symptoms and signs.

T

Tangential thinking (2) – A form of disorganized thinking in which one idea connects to the next, but the thoughts become confusing because they go off on a tangent and end on a different subject. The patient starts talking about one topic, but switches topics frequently and never gets back to the first topic.

Tardive dyskinesia (TD) (6) – TD is an adverse event that develops after extended periods (months, years, or decades) of taking conventional antipsychotics. TD consists of abnormal, involuntary movements. These movements often involve the mouth (chewing or puckering movements), the fingers or toes, or the trunk (such as rocking or swaying).

Therapy groups (7) – Therapy groups are a type of group therapy that focuses on helping patients explore on their relationships, their coping styles, and stressors that may make their symptoms worse. Rather than learning about symptoms and treatments only, patients work on the parts of their own personality styles that may interfere with psychosocial success.

Thought blocking (2) – A symptom of psychosis in which there is an interruption in the train of thought and the patient cannot put his or her thoughts into words. The thoughts are "blocked" from coming out. The person may be very slow to respond to questions or may not be able to respond at all.

Trade name (6) – A trade name is one of two names of a medicine. For example, Tylenol is a trade name for acetaminophen. All medicines have both a trade name and a generic name.

Treatment-refractory psychosis (6) – Patients with treatment-refractory psychosis have psychotic symptoms that have not cleared up even after trying several different antipsychotic medicines. Clozapine, one of the atypical antipsychotics, is more helpful than other medicines for treatment-refractory psychosis.

V

Vocational rehabilitation (7) – Vocational rehabilitation programs provide a variety of services, including vocational counseling and guidance, assessment of work skills and interests, training in particular job skills, support services (like transportation or interpreters), and assistance with job placement. These programs help individuals with psychosis find and keep jobs.

Voluntary inpatient treatment (5) – In the case of voluntary inpatient treatment, the patient chooses willingly to sign into the hospital. Also known as voluntary hospitalization.

W

Weight gain (6) – Weight gain is one of the side effects that may happen when taking some of the atypical antipsychotics.

Working diagnosis (3) – Mental health professionals use a working diagnosis to guide treatment planning before they have decided on a final diagnosis.

References

Albiston, D.J., Francey, S.M., & Harrigan, S.M. (1998). Group programmes for recovery from early psychosis. *British Journal of Psychiatry, 172*(33s), 117–121.

American Psychiatric Association. (2000). *Diagnostic and statistical manual of mental disorders*, 4th ed, text revision. Washington, DC: American Psychiatric Association.

American Psychiatric Association. (2004). *Practice guideline for the treatment of patients with schizophrenia.* 2nd ed. Arlington (VA): American Psychiatric Association; 2004 Feb. 114 p.

Birchwood M., Todd, P., & Jackson, C. (1998). Early intervention in psychosis. The critical period hypothesis. *British Journal of Psychiatry, 172*(33s), 53–59.

Bradford, D.W., Perkins, D.O., & Lieberman, J.A. (2003). Pharmacological management of first-episode schizophrenia and related nonaffective psychoses. *Drugs, 63*(21), 2265–2283.

Broome, M.R., Woolley, J.B., Tabraham, P., Johns, L.C., Bramon, E., Murray, G.K., et al. (2005). What causes the onset of psychosis? *Schizophrenia Research, 79*, 23–34.

Buckley, P.F. (2008). Factors that influence treatment success in schizophrenia. *Journal of Clinical Psychiatry, 69*(suppl 3), 4–10.

Edwards J., Harris M.G., & Bapat S. (2005). Developing services for first-episode psychosis and the critical period. *British Journal of Psychiatry, 48*, s91–97.

Edwards, J., & McGorry, P.D. (2002). *Implementing early intervention in psychosis: A guide to establishing early psychosis services.* London: Martin Dunitz.

Ehmann, M., MacEwan, G.W., & Honer, W.G. (Eds.) (2004). *Best care in early psychosis intervention: Global perspectives.* Oxon, UK: Taylor & Francis Group.

Goff, D.C. (2002). A 23-year old man with schizophrenia. *JAMA, 287*(24), 3249–3257.

Herz, M.I., & Marder, S.R. (2002). *Schizophrenia: Comprehensive treatment and management.* Philadelphia: Lippincott Williams & Wilkins.

International clinical practice guidelines for early psychosis. (2005). *British Journal of Psychiatry, 187,* s120–s124.

Kahn, R.S., Fleischhacker, W.W., Boter, H., Davidson, M., Vergouwe, Y., Keet, I.P.M., et al. Effectiveness of antipsychotic drugs in first-episode schizophrenia and schizoprheniform disorder: An open randomized clinical trial. *The Lancet, 371,* 1085–1097.

Langlands, R.L., Jorm, A.F., Kelly, C.M., & Kitchener, B.A. (2008) First aid recommendations for psychosis: Using the Delphi method to gain consensus between mental health consumers, carers and clinicians. *Schizophrenia Bulletin,* 34(3), 435–443.

Lieberman, J.A., Stroup, T.S., McEvoy, J.P., Swartz, M.S., Rosenheck, R.A., Perkins, D.O., et al. (2005). Effectiveness of antipsychotic drugs in patients with chronic schizophrenia. *New England Journal of Medicine, 353*(12), 1209–1223.

Lieberman, J.A., Stroup, T.S., & Perkins, D.O. (Eds.) (2006). *The American psychiatric publishing textbook of schizophrenia.* Arlington (VA): American Psychiatric Publishing.

Mallarkey, G. (Ed.) (1999). *Managing schizophrenia.* Hong Kong: Adis International.

McEvoy, J.P., Lieberman, J.A., Perkins, D.O., Hamer, R.M., Gu, H., Lazarus, A., et al. (2007). Efficacy and tolerability of olanzapine, quetiapine and risperdone in the treatment of early psychosis: A randomized, double-blind 52-week comparison. *American Journal of Psychiatry, 164*(7), 1050–1060.

Miller, T., Mednick, S.A., McGlashan, T.H., Libiger, J., & Johannessen, J.O. (Eds.) (2001). *Early interventions in psychotic disorders.* Dordrecht, The Netherlands: Kluwer Academic Publishers.

Mueser, K.T. & McGurk, S.R. (2004). Schizophrenia. *The Lancet, 363,* 2063–2072.

Penn, D.L., Wahdheter, E.J., Perkins, D.O., Mueser, K.T., Lieberman, J.A. (2005). Psychosocial treatment for first-episode psychosis: A research update. *American Journal of Psychiatry, 162,* 2220–2232.

Perkins, D.O., Hongbin, G., Weiden, P.J., McEvoy, J.P., Hamer, R.M., & Lieberman, J.A. (2008). Predictors of treatment discontinuation and medication nonadherence in patients recovering from a first episode of schizophrenia, schizophreniform disorder, or schizoaffective disorder: A randomized, double-blind, flexible-dose, multicenter study. *Journal of Clinical Psychiatry,* 69(1), 106–113.

Perkins, D.O., Leserman, J., Jarskog, L.F., Graham, K., Kazmer J., Lieberman, J.A. (2000). Characterizing and dating the onset of symptoms in psychotic illness: The Symptom Onset in Schizophrenia (SOS) inventory. *Schizophrenia Research*, 44, 1–10.

Saddicha, S., Manjunatha, N., Ameen, S., & Akhtar, S. (2008). Metabolic syndrome in first episode schizophrenia – A randomized double-blind controlled, short-term prospective study. *Schizophrenia Research, 101*, 266–272.

Sharma, T., Harvey, P.D. (2006). *The early course of schizophrenia.* Oxford, UK: Oxford University Press.

Stahl, M.S. (1999). *Psychopharmacology of antipsychotics.* London: Martin Dunitz.

Tandon, R., Belmaker, R.H., Gattaz, W.F., Lopez-Ibor Jr., J.J., Okasha, A., Singh, B., et al. (2007). World psychiatric association pharmacopsychiatry section statement on comparative effectiveness of antipsychotics in schizophrenia. *Schizophrenia Research, 100*, 20–38.

Tandon, R., Keshavan, M.S., & Nasrallah, H.A. (2008). Schizophrenia, "just the facts": What we know in 2008. Part 1: Overview. *Schizophrenia Research, 100*, 4–19.

Tandon, R., Targum, S.D., Nasrallah, H.A., & Ross, R. (2006). Strategies for maximizing clinical effectiveness in the treatment of schizophrenia. *Journal of Psychiatric Practice, 12*(6), 348–363.

The roadmap for antipsychotic psychopharmacology: An overview. (2007). *Journal of Clinical Psychiatry, 68*(11), 1799–1806.

U.S. Department of Health and Human Services (2006). *National consensus statement on mental health recovery.* Rockville (MD). U.S. Department of Health and Human Services: Substance Abuse and Mental Health Services Administration, Center for Mental Health Services, National Institutes of Health, National Institute of Mental Health.

Weiden, P.J., Scheifler, P.L., Diamond, R.J., & Ross, R. (1999). *Breakthroughs in antipsychotic medications: A guide for consumers, families, and clinicians.* New York: W.W. Norton & Company.

Zipursky, R.B., & Schulz, S.C. (Eds.) (2002). *The early stages of schizophrenia.* Washington (DC): American Psychiatric Publishing.

Index